# Juicing for Weight Loss

# 3 in 1 Bundle

# This book Includes: Alkaline Ketogenic Juicing, Celery Juice Recipes That Don't Taste Gross and Paleo Drinks

By Elena Garcia

Copyright Elena Garcia © 2019-2021

All rights reserved. No part of this publication may be reproduced, stored in a retrieval system, or transmitted, in any form or by any means, electronic, mechanical, photocopying, recording or otherwise, without the prior written permission of the author and the publishers.

The scanning, uploading, and distribution of this book via the Internet or via any other means without the permission of the author are illegal and punishable by law. Please purchase only authorized electronic editions, and do not participate in or encourage electronic piracy of copyrighted materials.

ISBN: 978-1-80095-065-8

**Disclaimer**

A physician has not written the information in this book. It is advisable that you visit a qualified dietician so that you can obtain a highly personalized treatment for your case, especially if you want to lose weight effectively. This book is for informational and educational purposes only and is not intended for medical purposes. Please consult your physician before making any drastic changes to your diet.

All information in this book has been carefully researched and checked for factual accuracy. However, the author and publishers make no warranty, expressed or implied, that the information contained herein is appropriate for every individual, situation or purpose, and assume no responsibility for errors or omission. The reader assumes the risk, and full responsibility for all actions and the author will not be held liable for any loss or damage, whether consequential, incidental, and special or otherwise, that may result from the information presented in this publication.

The book is not intended to provide medical advice or to take the place of medical advice and treatment from your personal physician. Readers are advised to consult their own doctors or other qualified health professionals regarding the treatment of medical conditions. The author shall not be held liable or responsible for any misunderstanding or misuse of the information contained in this book. The information is not intended to diagnose, treat, or cure any disease.

If you suffer from any medical condition, are pregnant, lactating, or on medication, be sure to talk to your doctor before making any drastic changes in your diet and lifestyle.

# Contents

Part 1 – Book 1 .................................................................................................................. 13

Alkaline Ketogenic Juicing .............................................................................................. 13

*Nutrient-Packed, Alkaline-Keto Juice Recipes for Balance, Energy, Holistic Health, and Natural Weight Loss* ........................................................................................................... 13

Introduction ..................................................................................................................... 15

Alkaline Keto Juices- Food Lists ..................................................................................... 21

    Recommended Alkaline Keto Fruit ............................................................................. 21

    Recommended Alkaline Keto Greens ........................................................................ 21

    Alkaline Keto Friendly Vegetables .............................................................................. 24

    Alkaline Keto Spices & Herbs for Your Juices ........................................................... 25

    Alkaline Keto Sweeteners and Supplements (Optional) ............................................ 26

    Alkaline Keto Fats ....................................................................................................... 27

    Alkaline Keto Friendly Milk & Other Liquids to Use in Your Juices ........................... 28

Why Alkaline Ketogenic Juices? How Can They Help You? ......................................... 29

What Is the Keto Diet? .................................................................................................... 31

What Is the Alkaline Diet? ............................................................................................... 32

Combining Alkaline with Keto ........................................................................................ 39

About the Recipes-Measurements Used in the Recipes .............................................. 41

Alkaline Keto Juice Recipes to Help You Thrive! .......................................................... 42

    Avocado Oil Green Juice for Energy & Weight Loss ................................................. 43

    No More Sugar Cravings Juice ................................................................................... 44

    Beautiful Skin Juice ..................................................................................................... 45

    Lemon Digestion and Weight Loss Tonic .................................................................. 46

    Super Hydrating Weight Loss Juice ........................................................................... 47

    Soft Balance Green Juice ........................................................................................... 48

    On the Go Alkaline Keto Juice Shot (Liver Lover) ..................................................... 49

    Energy Replenishment Juice ...................................................................................... 50

    Red Cabbage Detox Juice .......................................................................................... 51

    Vitamin C Green Juice for Natural Energy & Weight Loss ........................................ 52

    Light Alkaline Keto Juice ............................................................................................. 53

- Apple Cider Antioxidant Juice for Optimal Energy ... 54
- Fat Burn Weight Loss Herbal Alkaline Keto Juice ... 56
- No More Insomnia Alkaline Keto Juice ... 57
- Pomegranate Avocado Anti-Sugar Cravings Juice ... 58
- Alkalizing Mojito Juice ... 59
- Cucumber Kale Weight Loss Juice ... 60
- Super Tasty Spinach Juice (Not Kidding!) ... 61
- Tomato Mediterranean Antioxidant Juice ... 62
- Simple Flavored Kale Juice ... 63
- Easy Light Green Juice ... 64
- Naturally Sweet Celery Juice ... 65
- Coconut Kale Energy Boosting Concoction ... 66
- Simple Chlorophyll Juice ... 67
- Green Tea Bullet Proof Vitamin C Juice ... 69
- A Restorative Antioxidant Non-Green Juice ... 72
- Veggie Lover Juice ... 73
- Delicious Color Juice ... 74
- Mixed Green Juice ... 75
- Sexy Aphrodisiac Green Juice ... 76
- Healing Ashwagandha Juice ... 77
- Mint Parsley Delight ... 78
- Creamy Turmeric Drink ... 79
- Lime Mint Alkaline Water ... 80
- Pomegranate Green Juice ... 81
- Coconut Flavored Veggie Juice ... 82

Part 2 -Book 2 ... 85

Celery Juice Recipes That Don't Taste Gross ... 85

*47 Healthy and Balanced Celery Juice Recipes for Beauty, Weight Loss and Energy* ... 85

Introduction – No More Celery Juice Hype ... 87

Juicing Recipes- Food Lists ... 91

- Recommended Fruit ... 91

- Other Fruit (in moderation) .................................................................................. 92
- Recommended Greens to Use in Your Juicing Recipes ........................................ 92
- Vegetables to Use in Your Juices: ...................................................................... 93
- Spices & Herbs for Your Juices ........................................................................... 94
- Natural Sweeteners and Supplements (Optional) ............................................. 95
- Good Fats ............................................................................................................ 96

About the Recipes-Measurements Used in the Recipes ............................................ 98

Celery Juice Recipes to Help You Thrive! ................................................................... 99

- Recipe#1 Avocado Oil Celery Juice for Energy & Weight Loss ........................ 100
- Recipe#2 Quit Sugar Cravings Juice ................................................................. 101
- Recipe#3 Celery Juice Glow .............................................................................. 102
- Recipe#4 Celery Immune Tonic ........................................................................ 103
- Recipe#5 Super Hydrating Weight Loss Juice .................................................. 104
- Recipe#6 Holistic Balance Celery Juice ............................................................ 105
- Recipe#7 On the Go Celery Juice Shot (Liver Lover) ....................................... 106
- Recipe#8 Easy Energy Reboot Juice ................................................................. 107
- Recipe#9 Aroma Detox Mix .............................................................................. 108
- Recipe#10 Vitamin C Celery Juice for Natural Energy & Weight Loss ............ 109
- Recipe#11 Light Alkaline Keto Juice ................................................................. 110
- Recipe#12 Apple Cider Antioxidant Juice for Optimal Energy ........................ 111
- Recipe#13 Herbal Weight Loss Juice ................................................................ 113
- Recipe#14 Sleep Well Celery Juice ................................................................... 114
- Recipe#15 Pomegranate Celery Anti-Sugar Cravings Juice ............................. 115
- Recipe#16 Alkalizing Mojito Juice .................................................................... 116
- Recipe #17 Cucumber Kale and Carrot Juice ................................................... 117
- Recipe #18 Flavored Celery Juice ..................................................................... 118
- Recipe #19 Watermelon Antioxidant Juice ...................................................... 119
- Recipe #20 Simple Apple Lemon Juice ............................................................. 120
- Recipe #21 Honeydew Melon Green Juice ...................................................... 121
- Recipe #22 Easy Celery Juice ............................................................................ 122
- Recipe #23 Coconut Celery Concoction .......................................................... 123

Recipe #24 Broccoli and Orange Juice ............................................................. 124

Recipe #25 Green Tea High Energy Juice .......................................................... 125

Recipe #26 A Beta Carotene Powerhouse .......................................................... 126

Recipe #27 A Restorative Antioxidant Juice ....................................................... 127

Recipe #28 Veggie Medley Juice ....................................................................... 128

Recipe #29 Coconut Flavored Antioxidant Juice ................................................ 129

Recipe #30 Mixed Green Juice .......................................................................... 130

Recipe #31 Tantalizing Green Juice .................................................................. 131

Recipe #32 Healing Carrot Juice ....................................................................... 132

Recipe #33 Cucumber's Delight ......................................................................... 133

Recipe #34 Turmeric Celery Juice ..................................................................... 134

Recipe #35 Pineapple Lime Mint Juice .............................................................. 135

Recipe #36 Antioxidant Nutrition Juice ............................................................. 136

Recipe #37 Coconut Flavored Green Juice ........................................................ 137

Recipe#38 Creamy, Anti-Inflammatory Breakfast Delight ................................. 138

Recipe#39 Get Energized Antioxidant Juice ..................................................... 139

Recipe#40 Green Balance Party Juice ............................................................... 140

Recipe#41 Delicious Creamy Beet Juice ........................................................... 141

Recipe#42 Spicy Green Celery Juice ................................................................. 142

Recipe #43 Gazpacho Celery Juice .................................................................... 143

Recipe #44 "Replenish Yourself" Juice .............................................................. 144

Recipe #45 "Red Pepper Detox" Juice ............................................................... 145

Recipe #46 "Liver Lover" Juice ......................................................................... 146

Recipe #47 Creamy Chia Juice .......................................................................... 147

Part 3- Book 3 ............................................................................................................ 149

Paleo Drinks .............................................................................................................. 149

*Delicious and Easy Paleo Drink* ............................................................................. 149

*Recipes for Natural Weight Loss and* .................................................................... 149

*A Healthy Lifestyle* ................................................................................................. 149

Introduction .............................................................................................................. 153

About the Recipes-Measurements Used in the Recipes ................................. 156

Part 1 Paleo Smoothie Recipes ..................................................................................................... 157

    Recipe #1 Banana Breakfast ........................................................................................................ 158

    Recipe #2 Berry Blaster ............................................................................................................... 159

    Recipe #3 Paleo Hunger Hunter Smoothie ................................................................................. 160

    Recipe #4 Veggie Medley ............................................................................................................ 161

    Recipe #5 Easy Snack Smoothie ................................................................................................. 162

    Recipe #6 Healing Energy in a Glass ........................................................................................... 163

    Recipe #7 Mental Energy Smoothie ........................................................................................... 164

    Recipe #8 Berry Antioxidant Weight Loss Smoothie ................................................................. 165

    Recipe #9 Mango Green Madness ............................................................................................. 166

    Recipe #10 Sweet Date Healing .................................................................................................. 167

    Recipe 11 Vegetable Desire ........................................................................................................ 168

    Recipe #12 Simple Cream Smoothie .......................................................................................... 169

    Recipe #13 Mango Protein Smoothie ........................................................................................ 170

    Recipe #14 Guava Smoothie ....................................................................................................... 171

    Recipe #15 Cucumber Hydrating Green Smoothie .................................................................... 172

    Recipe #16 Paleo Zucchini Zip .................................................................................................... 173

    Recipe #17 Watermelon Dream ................................................................................................. 174

    Recipe #18 Mediterranean Gazpacho Smoothness .................................................................. 175

    Recipe #19 Celery Citrus Snack .................................................................................................. 177

    Recipe #20 Kale Green Powder Cup ........................................................................................... 178

    Recipe #21 Delicious Baobab Smoothie .................................................................................... 179

    Recipe #22 Choco Power Brain Smoothie ................................................................................. 180

    Recipe #23 The Smashing Pumpkin .......................................................................................... 181

    Recipe #24 Greens Sneaker ........................................................................................................ 182

    Recipe #25 Berry Best ................................................................................................................. 183

    Recipe #26 Watermelon Berry Dream ...................................................................................... 184

    Recipe #27 Papaya Weight Loss Surprise .................................................................................. 185

    Recipe #28 Creamy Peach .......................................................................................................... 186

    Recipe #29 Vitamin C Orange Smoothie ................................................................................... 188

    Recipe #30 Creamy Spinach Beauty Smoothie ......................................................................... 189

Recipe 31 Cherish Celery ..................................................................................... 190

Recipe #32 Healthy Skin Smoothie ...................................................................... 191

Recipe #33 Simple Nutty Paleo Protein Smoothie ............................................... 192

Recipe #34 Creamy Ginger Smoothie .................................................................. 193

## Part 2 Juices .............................................................................................................. 194

Recipe #35 Cucumber Kale and Carrot Juice ...................................................... 195

Recipe #36 Flavored Spinach Juice ..................................................................... 196

Recipe #37 Watermelon Antioxidant Juice ........................................................... 197

Recipe #38 Simple Apple Lemon Juice ................................................................ 198

Recipe #39 Honeydew Melon Green Juice .......................................................... 199

Recipe #40 Easy Green Juice .............................................................................. 200

Recipe #41 Coconut Kale Concoction .................................................................. 201

Recipe #42 Broccoli and Orange Juice ................................................................ 202

Recipe #43 Green Tea High Energy Juice ........................................................... 203

Recipe #44 A Beta Carotene Powerhouse ........................................................... 204

Recipe #45 A Restorative Antioxidant Juice ......................................................... 205

Recipe #46 Veggie Medley Juice .......................................................................... 206

Recipe #47 Cabbage and Coconut Juice ............................................................. 207

Recipe #48 Mixed Green Juice ............................................................................. 208

Recipe #49 Tantalizing Green Juice ..................................................................... 209

Recipe #50 Healing Carrot Juice .......................................................................... 210

Recipe #51 Cucumber's Delight ........................................................................... 211

Recipe #52 Turmeric Green Juice ........................................................................ 212

Recipe #53 Pineapple Lime Mint Juice ................................................................. 213

Recipe #54 Orange Pomegranate Juice ............................................................... 214

Recipe #55 Coconut Flavored Green Juice .......................................................... 215

## Part 3 Teas and Herbal Infusions ............................................................................ 216

Recipe #56 Ginger and Turmeric Tea ................................................................... 217

Recipe #57 Easy Chili Tea .................................................................................... 218

Recipe #58 Cumin and Caraway Tea ................................................................... 219

Recipe #59 Spicy Chai Tea ................................................................................... 220

Recipe #60 Ashwagandha Tea ..................................................................................... 221

Recipe #61 Sleep Well Tea ......................................................................................... 222

Bonus Recipe: Easy Mediterranean Tea ..................................................................... 223

Bonus Recipe: Lime Refresher Ice Tea ....................................................................... 224

Final Words and Your Paleo Quick Start Guide ......................................................... 225

**Paleo Lifestyle Made Easy** ............................................................................................ 225

# Part 1 – Book 1

## Alkaline Ketogenic Juicing

*Nutrient-Packed, Alkaline-Keto Juice Recipes for Balance, Energy, Holistic Health, and Natural Weight Loss*

By Elena Garcia

Copyright Elena Garcia © 2019

# Introduction

Thank You for purchasing this book.
It means you are very serious about your health and wellbeing.

Whether your goal is to lose weight, enjoy more energy, or learn a few delicious healing juicing recipes- you have come to the right place. With this guide, you will learn the art of juicing the right way, the way that is good for you and supports your health and weight loss goals.

This recipe book is a practical guide designed for busy people who value their health and wellbeing. Alkaline Ketogenic juicing is super healthy, and it's compatible with low or no sugar diets as well as super low carb diets.

Enriching your diet with alkaline keto juice can help you:
1. Eliminate sugar cravings.
2. Start losing weight naturally.
3. Enjoy more energy and vibrant health.
4. Help your body heal naturally by giving it a myriad of nutrients to help it get back in balance it deserves.

<u>This guide is NOT designed as a juice fast.</u>
We recommend you follow a balanced, clean food diet with enough calories to meet your nutritional needs (you can check out the first book in the series called Alkaline Ketogenic Mix to learn delicious clean food, alkaline keto recipes you will never get bored with).

Then, add healthy alkaline keto juice on top of that, and you will be amazed by the results.

Unstoppable energy, healthy glow, feeling amazing. Everyone around you will want to know your secret. Not to mention feeling confident about your transformation and knowing you are treating your body with the respect it deserves!

To make it as doable and straightforward as possible:

1. We will cover the main differences between juicing and smoothies, and why juicing might be more helpful to help you reach some of your health, wellness, and fitness goals much faster.

2. Then, we will move onto the alkaline-keto shopping lists- so that you know what ingredients you need to focus on.

You can even start taking action right away, as you are reading this book. The ingredients are inexpensive and easy to find.

3. Then, I will guide you through straightforward explanations of the alkaline and keto diets, and how these two can be combined as well as the fantastic health and wellness benefits, you can experience by enriching your diet with nutrient-packed, low-carb, low-sugar alkaline keto juices.

4. Finally, I'll introduce you to my favorite alkaline-keto juicing recipes.

## Juicing vs. Smoothies?

What I really like about alkaline-keto juices is that unlike traditional fruit juices or processed juices, they don't use any high sugar fruit.

Healthy, balanced juicing must be done the right way.

Unfortunately, many people miss that point. It's not their fault at all. There is just so much misinformation out there.

You see, juicing is an incredible way to boost your energy levels. When you juice, you extract pure juice, and there is no fiber, and so that allows your digestive system to rest. All the nutrients get easily absorbed into your system, and your body doesn't need to do any "extra hours" to digest it. Hence the almost instant energy boost and natural high.

Since there is nothing to digest and with juicing you give your body a ton of nutrients, you naturally start experiencing more energy.

However, juicing must be done the right way. Otherwise, you can really mess up your health goals. For example, if you juice fruit that is high in sugar, you will only cause havoc in your body. With no fiber, it's pure sugar that gets absorbed to your system to start causing imbalance.

Fruit is OK, as a part of a balanced, clean food diet, but juicing fruit that is high in sugar is not good for you. That is why I am a fan of alkaline keto style of juicing. With this method of juicing, you focus on low-sugar or no sugar ingredients. Veggies and fruit that are low in sugar.

These are examples of fruits that are low in sugar: lemons, limes, grapefruits, tomatoes, pomegranates (more in the next section where we will scrutinize all the food lists).

Because of their low sugar and high mineral content, they are considered alkaline-forming fruits. Alkaline diet doesn't like sugar (keto diet is very similar in this regard). If you are new to the alkaline and keto diets, that is one of the most important lessons, and it can really help you revolutionize your health.

Years ago, I was very desperate to lose weight, always signing up for all kinds of fads. I also tried juicing, but it didn't work for me, because I wasn't taught to do it the right way.

First of all, juicing all the fancy fruit was getting very expensive. And, I couldn't lose weight, and my health and energy levels were deteriorating because of all the sweet sugar-packed fruit juice I was drinking.

That is why I am so passionate about writing this book. I want to show you the right way, the balanced approach. And I will mention it again, especially for you young females out there- please eat enough and don't starve yourself with juices.

The recipes in this book are not a meal replacement. Instead, use it as a delicious and nutritious drink to sip on during the day, in between your meals.

Ok, so now let's compare juicing to smoothies. As you already know, juices extract the healing elixirs while getting rid of the pulp. It works great if you need a quick, natural energy boost while giving your digestive system a rest. It also works great for people who, for whatever health reason, can't tolerate too much fiber in their food. For example, my mom, even though she likes smoothies, can't have too much of them because of her digestive issues. That is why she's more focused on juicing.

Personally, I love both. I am also a big fan of healthy smoothies. To learn more about the Alkaline Keto smoothies, I recommend you read the second book in the Alkaline Keto Diet series: *Alkaline Ketogenic Smoothies.*

Ok, now that I have praised juicing and got you all excited (that was good news actually), I also have some bad news for you...

Well, it's not really that bad...as they say no pain no gain, right?

Ok, so here it is...making juices is a bit more time-consuming than blending smoothies. And it may take a bit more time to clean up.

My recommendation is to schedule your juicing time, for example, 2-3 times a week. Be sure to "batch-juice." That way, one juicing session can cover your juicing for the following day as well. You can store your fresh juice in a fridge, for no more than 24 hours.

Also, as you keep juicing more and more, you will get faster and faster. Trust me on that one! You will soon be a juicing expert (well, maybe you already are, who knows?).

For my smoothies, I use Vitamix Blender (but any blender will do as long as it works). For juicing, I use another tool, a fantastic juicer called Omega juicer. I love their brand. When choosing a juicer, be sure to use a cold press juicer that can also handle juicing a ton of greens.

You can learn more about my juicing recommendations and tools to help you on your juicing journey on my website:

www.YourWellnessBooks.com/resources

Finally, the recipes, as well as "nutritional philosophies" contained in this book, are very flexible and open-minded. Anyone can benefit from them; they are not only for people who follow alkaline or keto diets. So, whether you are alkaline keto full-time, or merely part-time (you are looking for easy tips and recipes to improve your health), you have come to the right place! Everyone can benefit from the power of alkaline keto juicing.

The moment you decide to focus on the abundance of healthy foods, you will automatically start craving all the good stuff.

So, without any further ado, let's do this. I am so excited for You!

# Alkaline Keto Juices- Food Lists

### Recommended Alkaline Keto Fruit

Both alkaline, as well as ketogenic diets, encourage you to stay away from sugar, including fruit that is high in sugar.

However, low-sugar fruits are allowed, and there are many ways to make them taste delicious (the recipes will show you how):

**Alkaline Keto Approved Fruits:**
- Limes
- Lemons
- Grapefruits
- Avocado (yes, it's a fruit)
- Tomato (yea, it's a fruit)
- Pomegranate

The following fruit is allowed occasionally, in small amounts, to flavor, infuse, or garnish:
- Green apple (sparingly)
- Orange (also sparingly)

### Recommended Alkaline Keto Greens

Greens are very good for you, and if used correctly, they will taste really nice in your juices. Don't worry if you have never made any green juice before, or are not too sure how it will taste. The recipes contained in this book got you covered.

While it may be tough to eat 4 cucumbers, 2 cups of spinach, 3 zucchini's with 3 red bell peppers and a bunch of kale, it's easy to drink their nutrients. Adding some greens to your salads and smoothies is already a significant step forward. But...juicing greens is a real game changer! Trust me on that one.

All leafy greens are super alkaline and also compatible with keto diets:

- Spinach
- Kale
- Microgreens
- Swiss Chard
- Arugula
- Endive
- Romaine Lettuce

+ other fresh leafy greens and greens as well as:

- Parsley
- Mint
- Cilantro

I prefer fresh greens to green powders...but...whenever I go traveling, or I am really pressed for time, I use a delicious green powder blend called Organifi.

I also like to add it to my recipes as it makes my juices taste really nice while adding a ton of superfoods at the same time.

You can learn more about it and how I use it with my recipes on my website (treat it as an additional recommendation):

www.yourwellnessbooks.com/resources

## Alkaline Keto Friendly Vegetables

All fresh veggies are considered alkaline, and most of them are also keto because they are low in carbs and low in sugar. The juice recipes from this book also call for good fats (more on the good fats later) to create alkaline keto balance and use fats for energy, instead of carbs.

**So, these are the best alkaline – keto veggies to use in your juices:**

- Red bell pepper
- Green bell pepper
- Yellow bell pepper
- Zucchini
- Broccoli
- Asparagus
- Colliflower
- Garlic
- Cucumbers
- Radishes

## Alkaline Keto Spices & Herbs for Your Juices

The following herbs and spices will make your juices taste delicious.
They are also full of anti-inflammatory properties.

Again, since there are no sugars and no nasty carbs, the following herbs and spices are both alkaline and keto friendly.

- Cinnamon
- Himalaya Salt
- Curry
- Red Chili Powder
- Cumin
- Nutmeg
- Italian spices
- Oregano
- Rosemary
- Lavender
- Mint
- Chamomile
- Fennel
- Cilantro
- Moringa

## Alkaline Keto Sweeteners and Supplements (Optional)

Stevia (very helpful if you want to make a sweet juice without using sugar or sugar-containing foods or supplements)

- Green Powders, like Organifi
- Spirulina
- Chorella
- Matcha
- Moringa Powder
- Maca Powder
- Ashwagandha Powder

Again, these are all optional. However, if you are interested in learning more, please visit our private website where I share more complimentary info with my readers. I have listed my favorite brands, green powders, and other health supplements to help you save your time on research:

www.YourWellnessBooks.com/resources

## Alkaline Keto Fats

**Plant-Based**

(these are both alkaline and keto friendly)

- Olive oil (organic, cold-pressed)
- Avocado oil
- Hemp oil
- Flaxseed oil
- Coconut oil
- Sesame oil

(please note, there is no need to purchase all of them, one, or two is enough; my two favorites are coconut oil and olive oil)

**Animal Based**

(these are more keto than alkaline because the alkaline diet prefers plant-based products. However, they are OK to use on a balanced diet full of greens and veggies)

- Organic butter
- Fish oil

Still, for the purpose of this book, we will be focusing mostly on plant-based fats because they work much better for juicing recipes.

However, other books in this series:

*Book 1 – Alkaline Ketogenic Mix &*
*Book 2 – Alkaline Ketogenic Smoothies*

Also, call for animal fats in some recipes.

## Alkaline Keto Friendly Milk & Other Liquids to Use in Your Juices

While these are not the main ingredients, they do work really well for some recipes. For example, some juicing recipes may taste way too intense, and so it makes sense to mix them with some alkaline-keto friendly liquids. Also, mixing your juices with other alkaline-keto friendly liquids will make your juicing habits less expensive.

**Plant-Based**

(these are both alkaline and keto friendly)

- Almond milk
- Coconut milk
- Hazelnut milk
- Coconut water
- Herbal infusions
- Organic Apple Cider Vinegar

+ coffee and caffeine, in moderation (for example, you can combine your juice with a little bit of green tea or red tea).

# Why Alkaline Ketogenic Juices? How Can They Help You?

The problem is that most people eat way too many carbs and sugars. The temptations are everywhere, I know! To make it even worse, we eat processed carbs and sugars (pasta, candy, cakes, etc.). Most people find it hard to start their day without carbs and sugar.

Luckily, once you get into the alkaline ketogenic lifestyle, through adding some delicious low-carb, low sugar, high-fat juices into your diet, you will be able to experience a whole range of health and wellness benefits as well as possible prevention of many diseases.

**Low carb, low sugar diets are proven to:**
-manage your sugar levels, prevent diabetes
-normalize your hormones and auto-immune system
-improve your neurological health
-have even been used in clinical settings to prevent Alzheimer's, epilepsies, type 3 diabetes

Alkaline-Keto juicing is the healthiest method of juicing- you are giving your body an instant injection of nutrients. That allows you to enjoy more energy naturally, you no longer crave carbohydrates and sugars.

Most sugar cravings we experience happen because our body is not feeling nourished...It's calling for help- *please, feed me! I am still hungry. Yes, I know, you fed me with pizza, ice cream, and a milkshake and you have been drinking coffee all day. But I am still tired. Can you please feed me with something so that I can actually do my job? My job is to keep you healthy. My job is to burn fat. My job is to make you look and feel amazing. Just, please! Feed me with something that will help me, will ya?*

**Here are other benefits of aligning your dietary choices with an alkaline ketogenic-friendly way:**

-you will experience reduced hunger and reduced cravings

-you will be burning fat and reducing carbs and so normalizing your insulin levels

-you will protect your heart while raising the good cholesterol

-you will enjoy the anti-age benefits, as keto foods promote longevity and vitality (while nobody ever promised us we will live forever, by making a decision to stay healthy, we make sure that the time we are here on earth, we feel good and are vibrant).

**Your transformation starts right here, right now.**

Alkaline Keto juices are one of the best and easiest tools to help you get started, even if you are new to living a healthy lifestyle.

**Now, let's have a look at:**

1. What the keto diet actually is.
2. What the alkaline diet is.
3. How these two can be successfully combined for optimal benefits while respecting your nutritional lifestyle choices and preferences.

The goal of this book is simple- I don't want to "push" any specific kind of a diet bandwagon or make you feel bad for eating a certain way.

Making people feel bad or fear-based marketing tactics never lead to any long-term transformation. Unfortunately, this is how most of the nutrition- health and fitness industry operates- fear-based marketing tactics and making people feel bad.

Instead, I want to inspire you and give you simple, healthy, and delicious tools (alkaline ketogenic juices) to help you get closer to your health, wellness, and fitness goals every day.

How about setting one simple goal, to begin with? Drink 1 alkaline ketogenic juice a day? Take meaningful I and inspired action from a place of curiosity and empowerment, not fear.

*Forget about perfection and focus on progress...*

We are very, very close to help you get started. In fact, if you have already read my book *Alkaline Ketogenic Mix*, or *Alkaline Diet for Weight Loss and Wellness*, or *Alkaline Paleo Mix*, feel free to skip the following section and dive right into the recipes.

What really matters here is practice. But a little bit of inspiring information and learning more about our amazing bodies can also help.

So...

## What Is the Keto Diet?

The simplest definition is:
**The ketogenic diet is a diet low in carbs and high in healthy fats.**
*It encourages to massively reduce the carbohydrate intake and replace it with good, healthy fats (more on healthy vs. unhealthy fats later). This cutback in carbs puts your body into a metabolic state called ketosis.*
*When in ketosis, your body becomes super-efficient at burning fat for energy. A ketogenic diet can also help reduce blood sugar and insulin levels.*

The fact is that we are designed to have periods where we "fast from carbs" and when our glucose levels are depleted.

Then, we start using our body very cleverly, using ketones for fuel. Ketones are the result of our body burning fat for food. The liver converts body fats and ingested fats into ketones.

*Transition your diet into a more keto-friendly diet, it's straightforward. It means fewer sugars and carbs and more good fats while eating well!*

Following this simple rule (even without going keto full-time) will help you transform your health. It will also help you lose weight naturally if you stay committed to it.

*You will no longer be hooked on all those "crappy carbs" and with the new "keto energy" you will feel much more motivated to work out and be more active.*

**So, here's what the ketogenic diet consists of:**
-75%- 80% fat (don't worry, it's all good fat and will not make you fat).
-5-15% healthy, clean protein
-5% good, unprocessed carbs (yea, you can still eat some carbs and the carbs we will be focusing on, will be healthy unprocessed no sugar carbs so no worries, there is no starvation involved here).

## What Is the Alkaline Diet?

"Going green" is the way to describe an alkaline diet and lifestyle because the focus is on green vegetables in general, as they are the most alkaline food you can ingest.
The benefits of the alkaline diet are numerous. Let us name a few:

**WEIGHT LOSS**

An alkaline diet will assist you in losing weight. One way that it does this is obvious. The foods you will be eating are very healthy, rich in minerals and low calorie in general.

You will also be reducing the amount of acid in your body. The body stores fat to protect itself from an abundance of acid. It is a self-preservation method. This is part of the reason why people who exercise a lot and drink an excess of caffeine cannot seem to lose those extra pounds. Their bodies are clinging to that fat to minimize the effects of all of the acid in their systems. Caffeine is really acid-forming, and it's not the most sustainable source of energy. That is why we recommend you drink it in moderation, for your own occasional enjoyment rather than a source of energy you depend on.

Another benefit of an alkaline lifestyle regarding weight loss is that alkaline systems have more oxygen in their cells. Oxygen is a very essential part of eliminating fat cells from the body. The more oxygen in your system, the more efficient your metabolism will be.

**ENERGY**

Going green does not only give you energy for the apparent reason that you are eating many more healthy, energizing vitamins. You are negating the acid-induced lethargy that is brought on by an unhealthy acid-forming diet.

Not only do our bodies need an abundance of oxygen to lose weight, but we also need oxygen in our cells to energize us. The lack of oxygen in our cells causes fatigue. No, it is not just because you worked too late or partied to hard the night before. It is internal. If your cells are trying to function in a highly acidic environment, they will not be able to transfer oxygen efficiently; leading of course to exhaustion.

Cells in the body also make something that is called adenosine triphosphate (ATP). If your system is very acidic, it harms the ability of your cells to produce it. In the scientific world, it is known as the "energy currency of life." The ATP molecule contains the energy that we need to accomplish most things that we do (both internally and externally).

## BODILY FUNCTIONS

Another benefit of the alkaline lifestyle is that your body will be able to function at an optimum level instead of being inhibited by acids:

- Your heartbeat is thrown off by acidic wastes in the body. The stomach suffers greatly from over-acidity.
- The liver's job is to get rid of acid toxins, but also to produce alkaline enzymes. By simply reducing your acid intake, you can internally boost your alkalinity thanks to your liver!
- Your pancreas thrives on alkalinity. Too much acid in your system throws off your pancreas. If you eat alkaline foods, your pancreas can regulate your blood sugars.
- Your kidneys also help to keep your body alkaline. When they are overwhelmed by an acidic diet, they cannot do their job
- The lymph fluids function most efficiently in an alkaline system. They remove acid waste. Acidic systems not only have a slower lymph flow causing acids to be stored; they can also cause acids to be reabsorbed through lymphatic ducts in your intestines that would typically be excreted.

## MENTAL FOCUS

The alkalinity of the system is one of the best ways to focus and strengthen the mind. Just as the rest of the body is poorly affected by acid-forming foods and other toxins, so is your brain. And as we all know, it should be possible to control your emotions and decision making with your mind. Guess what? If your body is too acidic and is not alkaline, your mental clarity will be cloudy, your decision making could be off, as well as your emotional state.

**DETOX**

Another huge benefit of an alkaline lifestyle is detoxification. First, you are going to be cutting out processed foods that are continually adding toxins to your system.

Secondly, you are going to be eating foods that allow your body to detox and rid itself of the acids that have built up in your system all this time. When we detoxify our bodies, our emotions, bodily functions, and mental functions can operate at their optimum levels.

The number of benefits that come with living alkaline are numerous. As you help your body rebalance its optimal blood pH, you will find, as we did, that you have never felt better. We are still seeing improvement and reaping the rewards of this holistic approach to not only eating alkaline foods but living alkaline.

Alkaline vs. Acidic? Sounds like the title fight for a lightweight boxing match. In reality, it is a fight, a fight for the pH balance of your body. pH levels are basically the measure of how acidic a liquid is.

*Our bodies function optimally when our blood is at about 7.35 -7.45 pH.*
pH levels range from 0 to 14. 0 is the highest level of acidity, but basically, everything 0-7 would be considered acidic. The 7-14 range is alkaline.

**Before we dive into complicated pH discussions, here is one thing to understand:**

-The alkaline <u>diet is not about changing or "raising" your pH</u>. This is where many alkaline guides go wrong. You see, our body is smart enough to **<u>self-regulate</u>** our pH for us, no matter what we eat.

Unfortunately, when you constantly bombard your body with acid-forming foods (for example processed foods, fast food, alcohol, sugar, crappy carbs, and even too much meat) you torture your body with incredible stress. Why? Well because it has to work harder to maintain that optimal pH...

Here's simple example...

Imagine you immerse yourself in a bath filled with ice. You say, but hey, my body can self-regulate its optimal temperature, right? And yes, it can. But it will eventually collapse, and you will get ill. The same happens with nutrition and our blood pH.

You can spend years indulging in toxic, processed, acid-forming foods that only deprive your body of its vital nutrients, saying: "But hey, my body will self-regulate its optimal blood pH."

And again, it will...but sooner or later it will give up and manifest a disease. It will accumulate fat as its natural defense function to protect your body from over-acidity. We don't wanna end up there, right?

So, to sum up- the alkaline diet is a natural, holistic system, a nutritional lifestyle that advocates the consumption of fresh, unprocessed foods that are rich in nutrients. These are called alkaline foods, and they help your body stimulate its optimal healing functions. Yes! A healthy body needs nutrients, and fresh fruits and vegetables are great for that.

The problem is that nowadays, most diets are filled with acid-forming foods that eventually make it hard for the body to regulate its optimal, healthy blood pH. Acidosis is very common in this day and age thanks to things we drink as well: coffee, alcohol, sugar, crappy carbs, and sodas all have an acidic effect on our bodies. Not to mention the chemicals many people take in through things like smoking and drugs (even prescription drugs have this effect).

There are many ways that you could become acidic. Eating acid-forming foods, stress, taking in too many toxins, and bodily processes all cause acidity in the body. Our internal systems try to balance themselves out and bring pH up with the help of alkaline minerals that we can ingest through our diet. If we do not take in a higher percentage of alkaline than acidic foods, we can become too acidic.

When you are acidic, it makes every process that your body does typically much more difficult or impossible for it to accomplish. We cannot absorb the beneficial nutrients we need from our food correctly. Our cells are not able to produce energy efficiently.

Our bodies are not able to fix damaged cells properly. We will not be able to detoxify properly. Fatigue and illness will drag you down. Sounds horrible; does it not? Here are some signs that you are overly acidic:

- ✓ Feeling tired all the time. You have no physical or mental drive at all.
- ✓ You always feel cold.
- ✓ You get sick easily.
- ✓ You are depressed or just feel "blah" all the time for no real reason
- ✓ You are easily overstimulated and stressed by noise, light, etc.
- ✓ You get headaches for no apparent reason
- ✓ You get watery eyes or inflamed eyelids.
- ✓ Your teeth are sensitive and may crack or chip
- ✓ Your gums are inflamed, and you are susceptible to canker sores
- ✓ You have recurring bouts with throat problems including tonsillitis
- ✓ Acidic stomach with acid indigestion and reflux is always an issue
- ✓ Your fingernails crack, split, and break
- ✓ You have super dry hair that sheds and is hay-like with split ends
- ✓ You have dry, ashy skin

- ✓ Your skin breaks out in acne or is irritated when you sweat
- ✓ You get leg cramps and spasms (this includes restless leg syndrome).

Changing your diet to one that is full of alkaline foods is one of the easiest and best things you can do for your overall health. I was so ecstatic that I did! And the best thing is- we will be combining alkaline foods with keto friendly meals to make it easy, delicious and fun! Much simpler to follow for the long term.

But the way we see it is this- it's perfect! Plus, it's not a diet, it's a lifestyle.
What I really like about the alkaline diet is that you don't have to be 100% perfect. It's enough to make sure you add a ton of greens and veggies and make your diet rich in alkaline foods.

It's easy to do when you focus on serving your lunch or dinner with a big green salad or start drinking alkaline keto smoothies and juices.

When it comes to the alkaline diet, there is something called the 70/30 rule meaning that about 70% of your diet should be fresh, nutrient dense alkaline-forming foods and the remaining 30% can be acid- forming foods (however they still should be clean and organic, for example, grass-fed meat or organic eggs).

**The common mistakes with the ketogenic diets:**
The most common mistake that people make is that they do not include enough veggies with their keto animal-based foods. That can cause imbalance and acidity. Hence, I am such a big fan of keto and alkaline diets combined together. Green vegetables are a fantastic addition to your keto diet.

They will help you have more energy and also add more variety to your diet. Alkaline Keto juicing is a simple to follow, natural tool to help you drink more vegetables. For many people, drinking veggies is actually easier than eating them.

The real keto lifestyle is about variety, abundance, and energy. It's hard to be successful with a keto diet if a menu consists entirely of animal products.

## Combining Alkaline with Keto

As surprising as it may sound, the ketogenic diet is actually pretty close to the alkaline diet.

The primary common rule is:
*Eat real food, eat clean food. Relax. Reduce stress. Enjoy the nature...*

**And these are the alkaline-keto guidelines to help you create vibrant health and energy:**

-add a lot of greens (one of the best ways is through the alkaline keto juices)
-add lots of healthy fats like omega 3 and saturated fats (again, alkaline keto juices will help you do that too)
-eat fresh, unrefined, natural foods
-get rid of processed carbs
-reduce fruit that is high in sugar (the recipes contained in this book only use low sugar fruit, and other fruit is used very sparingly, in small amounts, just to taste)
-eliminate gluten and sugar-containing foods and drinks
-get rid of refined oils

-consume moderate healthy protein (alkaline diet focuses more on plant-based protein; however, some quality plant-based protein is also OK on this diet as long as you add in a ton of greens and veggies; similarly, while the keto diet is mostly known for recommending animal-based protein, plant-based protein from leafy greens, nuts and seeds is also keto-friendly).

The alkaline keto diet can be created in different versions.

Listen to your body and give it what it needs to thrive.

## About the Recipes-Measurements Used in the Recipes

The cup measurement I use is the American Cup measurement.

I also use it for dry ingredients. If you are new to it, let me help you:

If you don't have American Cup measures, just use a metric or imperial liquid measuring jug and fill your jug with your ingredient to the corresponding level. Here's how to go about it:
*1 American Cup= 250ml= 8 Fl.oz.*

For example:

If a recipe calls for 1 cup of almonds, simply place your almonds into your measuring jug until it reaches the 250 ml/8oz marks.

I hope you found it helpful. I know that different countries use different measurements, and I wanted to make things simple for you. I have also noticed that very often those who are used to American Cup measurements complain about metric measurements and vice versa. However, if you apply what I have just explained, you will find it easy to use both.

# Alkaline Keto Juice Recipes to Help You Thrive!

*The golden rule is- when juicing, focus on:*

*-all kinds of veggies and greens that can be juiced*

*-low sugar fruit (for example lemons, limes, pomegranates, grapefruits)*

**Tips for getting started with juicing:**

- Prepare your house: Clean out the fridge and pantry and be sure it's stocked with tons of fresh and frozen produce.
- Begin by adding a handful or so of organic baby spinach into your juices, especially if you're new to green juices.
- Invest in a good juicer and set an intention (for example: "I can't wait to get started on this journey and to juice 3 times a week" – is a simple to follow through goal and intention).
- Prepare all your juices the night before and store them in air-tight containers for the following day. Making all the juices at once can save time in clean up and ensures you're ready with fresh juice whenever needed.
- There are so many variations of juicing, you can use the recipes and add or take away ingredients. Feel free to swap for your favorite ingredients, just make sure you're getting a tasty variety throughout the day.

Make sure you wash all the ingredients before you proceed to your juicing rituals.

Now, it's time for the recipes. I am so excited for you!

## Avocado Oil Green Juice for Energy & Weight Loss

Avocado oil offers good fat to help you absorb the minerals and vitamins from the juice. I love this juice whenever I need "an injection of energy." Himalaya salt adds alkaline minerals and makes this juice taste amazing. If you like spicy juices, feel free to add in some hot sauce, or chili powder.

**Servings: 2**

**Ingredients:**

- 1 lemon, peeled
- 1 lime, peeled
- 2 celery stalks, chopped
- a handful of arugula leaves
- 2 big cucumbers, peeled and chopped
- 2 tablespoons avocado oil
- Himalayan salt to taste
- Optional: A couple dashes of hot habanero sauce or chili powder

**Instructions:**

1. Place through a juicer.
2. Juice and combine with the avocado oil and Himalayan salt.
3. Serve in a glass and enjoy!

## No More Sugar Cravings Juice

This green juice recipe is beginner friendly, and it's also designed to help you fight sugar cravings.

The creamy consistency of this juice, micronutrients from green juice and super healthy fats from coconut oil will help you say no to sugar. Ginger adds anti-inflammatory properties.

**Serves: 2**

**Ingredients:**

- 1 cup spinach leaves
- 2-inch ginger, peeled
- 2 tablespoons melted coconut oil
- 1 cup of thick coconut milk
- Half teaspoon Ashwagandha
- Optional: stevia to sweeten

**Instructions:**

1. Place the spinach and ginger through a juicer.
2. Extract the juice, pour it in a big glass.
3. Combine with coconut milk and oil.
4. Add in the Ashwagandha.
5. Stir well and enjoy.

# Beautiful Skin Juice

This recipe is delicious and helpful for those who don't enjoy juicing greens. It also uses turmeric that is very alkalizing and also offers anti-inflammatory benefits.

When peeling, cutting and juicing turmeric, I recommend you use gloves (unless you want to walk around with orange nails and hands for the next 2 days lol).

**Servings: 2**

**Ingredients:**

- 2 big red bell peppers, chopped
- 1 big yellow bell pepper
- 2 inches of turmeric, peeled (use gloves)
- 2 lemons
- 2 tablespoons flax seed oil

**Instructions:**

1. Juice all the ingredients using a juicer.
2. Add in the flax seed oil.
3. Serve in a glass.
4. Enjoy!

## Lemon Digestion and Weight Loss Tonic

This recipe helps maintain a healthy digestive system and stimulate weight loss (thanks to grapefruits). It also makes your water taste great!

**Servings: 2**

**Ingredients:**

- 1 cup of mint leaves, chopped
- 1 grapefruit, peeled and chopped
- 1 lemon, peeled and halved
- 1 inch of ginger, peeled
- 1 cup of water
- Optional: stevia to sweeten

**Instructions:**

1. Place all the ingredients in a juicer. Juice.
2. Mix with water.
3. Serve chilled with some ice cubes.
4. Enjoy!

## Super Hydrating Weight Loss Juice

This simple recipe is another easy to follow option for those who don't enjoy juicing leafy greens. Cucumbers taste really delicious in juices and combine really well with coconut oil and milk.

**Servings: 2**

**Ingredients:**

- 4 big cucumbers, peeled and chopped
- 1 lime peeled and chopped
- 2 green bell peppers
- 2 tablespoons coconut oil, melted
- Himalaya salt to taste, if needed
- Half cup thick coconut milk

**Instructions:**

1. Place all the ingredients through a juicer.
2. Extract the juice.
3. Pour into a chilled glass.
4. Add in the coconut oil and coconut milk.
5. Taste with Himalaya salt if needed.
6. Enjoy!

## Soft Balance Green Juice

Celery juice offers anti-inflammatory properties and Vitamin C to help you enjoy more energy and take care of your immune system.

Maca powder is a fantastic hormone balancer, and I love using it with this juice. Red bell pepper makes it taste really delicious, and so does the cinnamon and nutmeg powder.

**Servings: 2**

**Ingredients:**

- 1 cup celery, chopped
- 1 inch of ginger, peeled
- 1 red bell pepper
- 2 tablespoons avocado oil
- half teaspoon cinnamon powder
- half teaspoon maca powder
- cinnamon and nutmeg powder to taste

**Instructions:**

1. Juice all the ingredients using a juicer.
2. Pour in a glass.
3. Add in the avocado oil, maca, cinnamon, and nutmeg powder.
4. Stir well, serve and enjoy!

## On the Go Alkaline Keto Juice Shot (Liver Lover)

This recipe is perfect if you are too busy to juice…

You know…setting up the juicer, cleaning up.

Well, this recipe doesn't even need a proper juicer. A simple lemon squeezer will do.

This simple recipe helps detoxify the liver, it works really well first thing in the morning.

**Serves: 1**

**Ingredients:**

- 2 lemons
- 1 tablespoon avocado oil or olive oil
- Pinch of Himalaya salt

**Instructions:**

1. Juice the lemons.
2. In a small glass, combine the lemon juice with the oil and Himalaya salt.
3. Stir well, say 3-2-1 and drink.
4. To your health!

(yea…sometimes it's about the taste, and sometimes it's about the benefit)

**Energy Replenishment Juice**

This recipe uses coconut water to help you spice up your green juice and make it taste amazing.

**Serves: 1-2**

**Ingredients:**

- 1 cup of coconut water
- 1 cup spinach leaves
- 1-inch ginger
- 1 grapefruit
- Ice cubes

**Instructions:**

1. Juice the spinach, ginger, and grapefruit.
2. Combine with coconut water and ice cubes.
3. Serve and enjoy!

## Red Cabbage Detox Juice

Cabbage is an excellent source of sulfur, which helps purify the blood and detoxify the liver. Fennel and mint help create a nice flavor while adding in more healing nutrients to help you thrive.

**Servings: 2**

**Ingredients:**

- 1 small red cabbage
- 1 fennel bulb
- A handful of mint leaves
- Half cup almond milk
- 2 tablespoons melted coconut oil
- Optional- stevia to sweeten

**Procedure:**

1. Juice all the ingredients.
2. Add the almond milk and coconut oil.
3. Stir well.
4. Enjoy!

## Vitamin C Green Juice for Natural Energy & Weight Loss

This simple juice recipe offers a fantastic combination of greens with alkaline keto friendly fruits and healthy fats. It will help you feel energized while eliminating sugar cravings.

Servings: 1-2

**Ingredients:**

- 2 grapefruits, peeled
- 1 cup kale leaves, chopped
- 1-inch ginger
- 2 tablespoon flax seed oil or sesame oil
- Optional: stevia to sweeten

**Instructions:**

1. Juice the grapefruits, kale leaves, and ginger.
2. Combine with flax seed oil (or sesame oil).
3. If needed, sweeten with stevia.
4. Serve and enjoy!

## Light Alkaline Keto Juice

This juice is particularly useful for healthy eyesight and beautiful skin as it is packed with Vitamins A and C.

It also helps fight inflammation and takes care of your liver.

**Ingredients:**

- 1 cup radish, cut into smaller pieces
- 1-inch ginger
- 1 lime, peeled
- 1 fennel bulb, cut into smaller pieces
- 1 tablespoon sesame or flax seed oil
- Pinch of Himalayan salt

**Instructions:**

1. Juice the radish, ginger, lime, and fennel.
2. Add in the Himalayan salt and oil.
3. Stir well, serve and enjoy!

## Apple Cider Antioxidant Juice for Optimal Energy

This recipe is full of miraculous nutrients to help you get rid of toxins. Its therapeutic properties are enhanced by Apple Cider Vinegar.

**Servings: 1-2**

**Ingredients:**

- 2 cucumbers, peeled and sliced
- Half cup of parsley leaves
- Half cup of mint leaves
- 2 tablespoons of olive oil
- 1 tablespoon apple cider vinegar (organic)
- Himalayan salt to taste (optional)

**Instructions:**

1. Juice all the ingredients.
2. Add in the olive oil, apple cider vinegar, Himalayan salt, and black pepper.
3. Serve and enjoy!

***To learn more about Apple Cider Vinegar (for health, home, and beauty), I highly recommend you read my book:

***Apple Cider Vinegar: The Miraculous Natural Remedy!: Holistic Solutions & Proven Healing Recipes for Health, Beauty, and Home***

If your goal is weight loss and body detoxification, you can start adding about 1-2 tablespoons (a day) of quality, organic, apple cider vinegar to your alkaline-keto drinks.

Apple cider vinegar goes really well with therapeutic alkaline keto juices (and also smoothies). It's inexpensive and very effective.

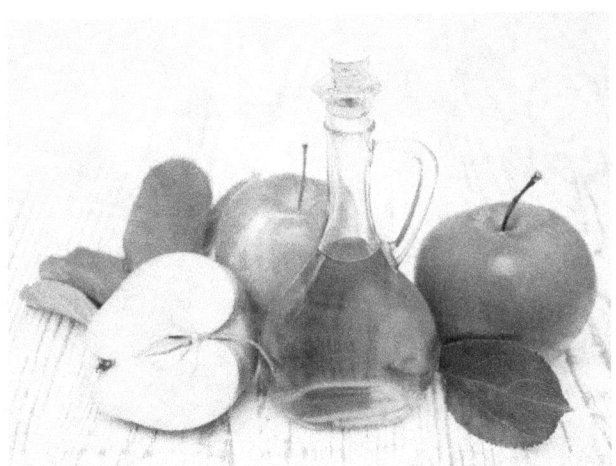

## Fat Burn Weight Loss Herbal Alkaline Keto Juice

This recipe fuses the low sugar alkaline fruits with horsetail infusion. Horsetail infusion is an excellent natural remedy to get rid of water retention, lose weight, and burn fat. It's full of alkaline minerals and blends really well with this juice.

**Ingredients:**

- A handful of fresh mint leaves
- 1 grapefruit, peeled
- 1 lime, peeled
- Half inch ginger, peeled
- 2 cucumbers, peeled
- Half cup horsetail infusion cooled down
- Optional: stevia to sweeten

**Instructions:**

1. First, juice all the ingredients.
2. Combine with horsetail infusion. Add stevia if needed.
3. Serve and enjoy!

# No More Insomnia Alkaline Keto Juice

This delicious herbal juice uses verbena- a herb used to stimulate relaxation and peace of mind.

**Servings: 1-2**

**Ingredients:**

- 1 cup verbena infusion, cooled down a bit (use 1 teabag per cup)
- 2 grapefruits, peeled and sliced
- 1 cup chopped celery
- A handful of fresh mint leaves
- Stevia to sweeten

**Procedure:**

1. Juice the grapefruits, celery, and mint leaves.
2. Mix the juice with the infusion.
3. Stir well and add stevia for naturally sweet taste.
4. Enjoy!

*Verbena is a pretty safe herb, but there is not enough information to confirm whether it can be used during pregnancy or breastfeeding. The same applies to possible contraindications with other medications. I always recommend consulting with your doctor first.*

## Pomegranate Avocado Anti-Sugar Cravings Juice

This recipe will help you get rid of sugar cravings while feeding your body with a myriad of nutrients it needs to thrive.

Pomegranate juice is full of alkaline minerals as well as Vitamin C.

It's a natural antioxidant and anti-inflammatory. It blends really well with ginger, turmeric, and mint. You can't juice avocado...but you can use avocado oil.

**Servings: 2**

**Ingredients:**

- 1 cup pomegranate seeds
- 1-inch ginger root, peeled
- 1-inch turmeric root, peeled
- A handful of fresh mint leaves
- 2 tablespoons of avocado oil
- Stevia to sweeten (optional)

**Procedure:**

1. Juice the pomegranate seeds, ginger, turmeric, and mint.
2. Combine with avocado oil.
3. Serve and enjoy!

## Alkalizing Mojito Juice

It's time for a simple and super healthy, non-alcoholic version of mojito!

**Servings: 2-3**

**Ingredients:**

- 1 cucumber, peeled and sliced
- Half cup fresh mint leaves
- 2 limes, peeled and sliced
- A few mint leaves to garnish
- A few lime slices to garnish
- 3 cups alkaline (or filtered) water
- Stevia to sweeten (optional)

**Instructions:**

1. Juice all the ingredients (except the mint and lime slices for garnishing)
2. Pour the fresh juice into a tall water jar or pitcher.
3. Add fresh water and ice cubes.
4. Now, add the mint leaves and lime slices.
5. Stir in well, chill in a fridge for a few hours, and serve.
6. Enjoy!

## Cucumber Kale Weight Loss Juice

While it's hard to eat a mountain of greens and cucumbers, it's easy to drink their juice and get all the vital nutrients from them. Avocado oil offers good fat to help you absorb the minerals and vitamins from the juice.

**Servings: 2**

**Ingredients:**

- 1 cup of kale, chopped
- 4 big cucumbers, peeled and chopped
- 2 limes, peeled
- 2 tablespoons of avocado oil
- Himalaya salt and black pepper to taste (optional)

**Instructions:**

1. Place through a juicer.
2. Pour into a glass and mix in some Himalayan salt and black pepper to taste. Stir in the avocado oil.
3. Enjoy!

## Super Tasty Spinach Juice (Not Kidding!)

While pure spinach juice can be a bit hardcore, this recipe is a bit different as it uses coconut milk and delicious spices...It's very nutritious and rich in good fats. And yes...you still get all the benefits of drinking green juice...

**Serves: 2**

**Ingredients:**

- 2 cups of fresh spinach leaves
- 2-inch ginger, peeled
- 1 cup almond milk, unsweetened
- 1 cup coconut milk, unsweetened
- 2 tablespoons coconut oil
- 1 teaspoon cinnamon powder
- Pinch of nutmeg powder
- Optional: stevia to sweeten

**Instructions:**

1. Place all the ingredients through a juicer.
2. Extract the juice, pour it in a big glass.
3. Add in some melted coconut oil, coconut and almond milk as well as spices and stevia.
4. Stir well and enjoy.

## Tomato Mediterranean Antioxidant Juice

Tomato, ginger, and good oils make an excellent combination. Mediterranean spices take it to the next level!

**Servings: 2**

**Ingredients:**

- 8 big organic tomatoes, chopped
- 2 inches of ginger, peeled
- 2 garlic cloves, peeled
- 2 tablespoons olive oil
- 2 tablespoons Mediterranean spices (oregano, thyme, rosemary- it's really up to you)
- Himalaya salt to taste

**Instructions:**

1. Juice all the ingredients using a juicer.
2. Combine with olive oil and spices.
3. Enjoy!

## Simple Flavored Kale Juice

While I definitely don't promote the idea of juicing sugary fruits, it's absolutely fine to add a bit of apple to your green juice to make it taste sweeter.

**Servings: 2**

**Ingredients:**
- 2 cups of kale, chopped
- 1 green apple, peeled and chopped
- 1 lemon, peeled and halved
- 1 inch of ginger, peeled
- 1-inch turmeric, peeled
- 1 tablespoon flaxseed oil
- 1 teaspoon cinnamon powder
- 1 teaspoon maca powder
- Optional: stevia to sweeten

**Instructions:**
1. Place all the ingredients in a juicer.
2. Juice, mix with flaxseed oil, maca, and cinnamon powder.
3. Serve in a glass.
4. If needed, sweeten with stevia.
5. Enjoy!

## Easy Light Green Juice

This is a super hydrating, alkalizing green juice with a nice, light flavor.

**Servings: 2**

**Ingredients:**

- 4 medium cucumbers, peeled and chopped
- 1 romaine lettuce
- 2 limes
- 2 tablespoons avocado oil
- Optional: Himalayan salt to taste

**Instructions:**

1. Place all the ingredients through a juicer.
2. Extract the juice.
3. Mix with avocado oil and Himalayan salt
4. Pour into a chilled glass and enjoy!

## Naturally Sweet Celery Juice

Red bell peppers are one of my favorite veggies to juice.

They are naturally sweet and full of vitamins and minerals.

They make any green juice taste amazing. This recipe is perfect for people who are just getting started on juicing celery and want to make a juice that feels nice.

**Servings: 2**

**Ingredients:**

- 1 cup celery, chopped
- 3 red bell peppers, chopped
- 1 inch of ginger, peeled
- 1 lime, peeled
- 1 cup water, filtered, preferably alkaline
- Mint leaves to garnish
- Optional: stevia to sweeten if needed

**Instructions:**

1. Juice all the ingredients using a juicer.
2. Pour in a big glass or a jar. Combine with water.
3. Stir well. Sweeten with stevia if needed.
4. Garnish with mint leaves.
5. Serve and enjoy!

## Coconut Kale Energy Boosting Concoction

Compared to other juicing recipes, this one is relatively simple and quick to make as it leverages the coconut water. Just perfect as a quick, energy-boosting juice. Great for those who are just getting started on green juice! Apple cider vinegar is an added bonus.

**Servings: 2**

**Ingredients:**

- 1 cup kale, chopped
- Half of green apple, peeled and chopped
- 1 cup of coconut water, unsweetened
- 1 tablespoon coconut oil
- 1 tablespoon apple cider vinegar
- 1 teaspoon cinnamon powder

**Instructions:**

1. Juice the kale and apple.
2. Pour into a glass and mix with 1 cup of coconut water.
3. Stir well, add in 1 teaspoon of cinnamon powder.
4. Stir again and add the coconut oil and apple cider vinegar.
5. Stir well again, serve and enjoy!

## Simple Chlorophyll Juice

This juice is great for boosting your energy and stimulating weight loss. Liquid chlorophyll is a fantastic way of enriching your juice with more nutrients, and it's perfect if you are too busy to juice the heaps of greens. To make this recipe, you don't even need an Omega Juicer, you could easily do with a simple lemon squeezer.

**Servings: 2**

**Ingredients:**

- 2 big grapefruits
- 1 cup thick coconut milk, full fat, unsweetened
- 1 tablespoon avocado oil
- Half teaspoon cinnamon powder
- A few drops of liquid chlorophyll
- Stevia to sweeten- optional

**Instructions:**

1. Juice the grapefruits (a lemon squeezer tool like the one on the picture below, will do for this recipe).
2. Combine the juice with avocado oil, coconut milk, cinnamon powder, and liquid chlorophyll.
3. Stir well, serve in a glass and enjoy!

A simple lemon squeezer tool like this one can be a real life-saver.

Perfect for simple juice recipes including limes, lemons, and grapefruits (healthy alkaline keto fruits!).

Simple to use and inexpensive! Be sure to purchase a lemon squeezer tool that is sharp enough to juice grapefruits as well.

Easy peasy lemon squeezy!

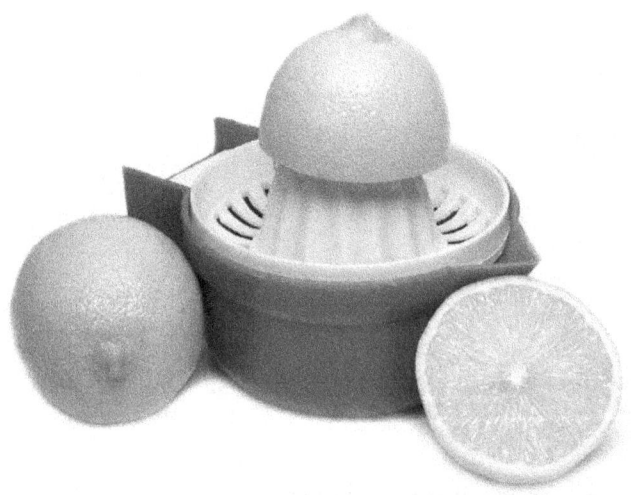

## Green Tea Bullet Proof Vitamin C Juice

This recipe uses green tea to help you boost your energy levels and burn fat. Ginger adds to anti-inflammatory properties. Then, there is grapefruit, super-rich in Vitamin C and alkaline minerals.

That mix combines really well with coconut oil. So tasty and good for you! Once again, for this recipe, you don't even need a fancy juicer. A simple lemon squeezer will do.

**Servings: 2**

**Ingredients:**

- 1 big grapefruit
- 1-inch ginger, peeled
- 1 cup green tea, cooled down (use 1 teabag per cup)
- 2 tablespoons coconut oil
- Stevia to sweeten if needed

**Instructions:**

1. Make the green tea, add in ginger, and leave covered to boil.
2. In the meantime, juice grapefruit using a lemon squeezer or a juicer.
3. In a small hand blender, combine the grapefruit juice and coconut oil. Process until smooth.
4. Once the green tea cools down, pour the juice into a big glass or a jar, and combine with the tea. Serve as it is or chilled. Enjoy!

**Grapefruit juice benefits:**

-helps in weight loss (it's low in calories and high in nutrients)

-very low in carbs and sugars

-stimulates the lymphatic system, helping you feel lighter and more energized

-boost the immune system

-Very alkalizing!

## Beta Carotene Powerhouse for Healthy-Looking Skin

This juice is a fantastic combination of tomatoes, turmeric, and ginger to help you have beautiful and healthy-looking skin while enjoying more energy without having to rely on caffeine.

**Servings: 2**

**Ingredients:**

- 6 big tomatoes, chopped
- 2-inch turmeric, peeled
- 2-inch ginger, peeled
- 2 tablespoons olive oil
- Pinch of Himalayan salt

**Instructions:**

1. Juice all the ingredients.
2. Pour into a glass and add in the olive oil and Himalayan salt.
3. Enjoy!

## A Restorative Antioxidant Non-Green Juice

This juice shows once again that healthy juicing can go beyond juicing greens. Tomatoes blend very well with grapefruits and ginger.

**Servings: 2**

**Ingredients:**

- 4 tomatoes, cut into smaller pieces
- 1-inch ginger, peeled
- 2 big grapefruits, peeled and cut into smaller pieces
- 2 tablespoons avocado oil

**Instructions:**

1. Juice all the ingredients.
2. Combine with avocado oil.
3. Serve in a big glass and enjoy!

## Veggie Lover Juice

*Elena? Why juicing? Why not just eat those veggies?*
My mom used to ask me this question all the time.

Well....would it be even possible to eat through a massive pile of veggies below? Juicing makes it easier. Think of all the micronutrients your body is getting in an easy to absorb "vitamin and mineral injection".

**Servings: 4**

**Ingredients:**

- 3 medium carrots, peeled and cut into smaller pieces
- 1 beet (with greens), peeled
- 4 large tomatoes, cut into smaller pieces
- 2 large handfuls spinach
- Half head cabbage, chopped
- 1 red bell pepper, chopped
- 1 large celery stalk, chopped
- A handful of mint leaves
- 4 tablespoons avocado oil

**Instructions:**

1. Juice all the ingredients.
2. Pour into a big jar, combine with avocado oil, serve in smaller glasses and enjoy!
3. If needed, season with some Himalaya salt.

## Delicious Color Juice

While pure green juice might be a bit too "hardcore" even for experienced juicing fanatics, it tastes amazing when mixed with other ingredients, such as red bell peppers. The color is amazing too!

**Servings: 2**

**Ingredients:**

- Half cabbage, chopped
- 4 red bell peppers, sliced
- 2 limes, peeled
- 2 tablespoons avocado oil

**Instructions:**

1. Juice all the ingredients.
2. Pour into a glass and mix with some avocado oil.
3. Enjoy!

## Mixed Green Juice

This recipe is great if you happen to have some arugula leaves leftovers and don't feel like going for another salad. And yes, arugula juice tastes amazing when mixed with other ingredients!

**Servings: 2**

**Ingredients:**

- 1 cup arugula leaves
- A few slices of green apple
- 1 lemon, peeled and cut into smaller pieces
- 1 tablespoon avocado oil

**Instructions:**

1. Place though a juicer.
2. Juice and pour into a glass or a small jar.
3. Stir in some avocado oil.
4. Enjoy!

## Sexy Aphrodisiac Green Juice

Once again, we are juicing arugula leaves while adding in some sweetness from red bell peppers and flavors from cilantro and mint.

Arugula is a super nourishing and hydrating leafy green. It's recommended for bone health and it also helps reduce inflammation in the body. Och…and it's an aphrodisiac too!

**Servings: 2**

**Ingredients:**

- 1 cup arugula leaves
- 2 red bell peppers, chopped
- 2 tablespoons fresh cilantro leaves
- 2 tablespoons fresh mint leaves
- 2 tablespoons avocado oil

**Instructions:**

1. Place all the ingredients though a juicer.
2. Juice and add in the avocado oil.
3. Serve and enjoy!

## Healing Ashwagandha Juice

Ashwagandha powder is a great choice to help you re-balance your energy levels while feeling more relaxed. Coconut milk makes this juice creamy and soft.

**Servings: 2**

**Ingredients:**

- 2 red bell peppers, chopped
- 1 lime, peeled and chopped
- 1 cup coconut milk
- 2 tablespoons coconut oil
- Half teaspoon Ashwagandha powder

**Instructions:**

1. Juice the bell peppers and a lime.
2. Pour into a small hand blender and combine with coconut milk, coconut oil and Ashwagandha.
3. Blend until smooth and creamy.
4. Pour into a glass and enjoy!

## Mint Parsley Delight

Parsley leaves add in a ton of vitamins and nutrients such as Vitamin A, Vitamin C and Iron. Mint helps in digestion and brings an amazing aroma to the table. Almond milk makes this juice even more nutritious (and creamy)!

**Servings: 2**

**Ingredients:**

- A handful of fresh mint leaves
- A handful of fresh parsley leaves
- 2 lemons, peeled and chopped
- 1 cup almond milk
- Stevia to sweeten, if needed
- 2 tablespoons avocado oil

**Instructions:**

1. Juice mint and parsley.
2. Pour into a glass or a small jar.
3. Add the almond milk, stevia and avocado oil.
4. Stir well and enjoy!

## Creamy Turmeric Drink

Turmeric is full of polyphenols that help well in weight loss.

It's a great addition to your juices and creates a nice, spicy aroma that is very easy to get hooked on.

I love combining this juice with full-fat, creamy coconut milk and cinnamon. So yummy, healthy, alkaline and keto!

**Servings: 2-3**

**Ingredients:**

- 3-inch turmeric, peeled
- 4 cucumbers, peeled and chopped
- 1 cup warm coconut milk
- 1 tablespoon coconut oil
- 1 teaspoon cinnamon

**Instructions:**

1. Heat up the coconut milk and add in the cinnamon and coconut oil.
2. Stir well and set aside.
3. In the meantime, juice the cucumbers and turmeric.
4. Add the fresh juice to the coconut milk concoction.
5. Stir well, serve and enjoy!

## Lime Mint Alkaline Water

This recipe uses fresh juice to make your water taste delicious!

**Servings: 3-4**

**Ingredients:**

- ¼ cup mint leaves, fresh
- 2 limes, peeled and chopped
- 4-inch ginger, peeled
- 4 big cucumbers, peeled and chopped
- 4 cups water, filtered, preferably alkaline
- Optional: stevia to sweeten if desired

**Instructions:**

1. Place the mint leaves, limes, ginger and cucumbers through a juicer.
2. Juice.
3. Pour into a big water jar and combine with 4 cups of filtered water.
4. Stir well, if needed sweeten with stevia.
5. Enjoy!

## Pomegranate Green Juice

With pomegranate, you are sure to enjoy a juice that is full of antioxidants and nutrients that are good for weight loss.

Oh, and we are sneaking in some greens too. Great way to make use of some salad leftovers! Some days, I really like to keep it simple.

**Servings: 2**

**Ingredients:**

- 1 cup pomegranate seeds
- 1 cup of mixed greens of your choice
- 2 tablespoons flaxseed oil

**Instructions:**

1. Juice the greens and pomegranates.
2. Pour into a glass and stir in the flaxseed oil.
3. Serve and enjoy!

## Coconut Flavored Veggie Juice

The juice ingredients are rich in phytonutrients and antioxidants.

Coconut oil makes this concoction taste really delicious, while helping you reduce sugar and carb cravings too.

Focus on adding greens and good oils and it will be so much easier to live a healthy lifestyle! This recipe proves just that.

**Servings: 2**

**Ingredients:**

- 1 cup kale, chopped
- 3 carrots, peeled
- 2 tablespoons coconut oil, melted
- 1 cup thick coconut milk
- Half teaspoon cinnamon powder to serve

**Instructions:**

1. Place the kale and carrots through a juicer.
2. Juice and pour into a glass.
3. Stir in the coconut oil and coconut milk.
4. Sprinkle over a bit of cinnamon powder.
5. Serve and enjoy!

**Bonus Recipe – Gluten-Free Pancakes Made with the Pulp**

You can use the pulp from your juices to make healthy, low-carb, gluten-free pancakes. The recipe below is a template that you can personalize depending on your taste preferences.

You can make sweet pancakes using stevia and using pulp from limes, lemons or pomegranates.

Vegetable pulp works better for spicy or savory pancakes.

**Ingredients:**

- 4 tablespoons pulp
- 1 teaspoon spices (depending on your taste preferences)
- 2 organic eggs
- 8 tablespoons almond flour
- 1 tablespoon coconut oil (for the mixture)
- 3 tablespoons coconut oil (for frying)

**Instructions:**

1. Heat up the coconut oil in a skillet (medium heat).
2. In the meantime, blend the pulp, eggs, flour and 1 tablespoon coconut oil, until smooth creamy mixture.
3. Form little pancakes and start frying on both sides.
4. Serve and enjoy!

**Let's finish this book with a few words of motivation and inspiration.**

It's all about taking meaningful and inspired action.

Ditch perfection for progress. Focus on daily micro steps. Healthy choices. Ask yourself- is this taking me closer to my goals?

Cultivate positive self-talk. Stop beating yourself up.

Beautiful results will start taking place.

Think where you will be 5 years from now…The baby steps will compound into a big transformation.

Be patient. Focus on the here and now.

Thank you again for reading.

I am really grateful for you,

Until next time,

Wishing you all the best on your journey,

Elena

www.YourWellnessBooks.com

## Part 2 -Book 2

## Celery Juice Recipes That Don't Taste Gross

*47 Healthy and Balanced Celery Juice Recipes for Beauty, Weight Loss and Energy*

By Elena Garcia

Copyright Elena Garcia © 2019

## Introduction – No More Celery Juice Hype

Yes, celery juice can be good for us, we have all heard it before.

But it can also be very harmful when overdone. And pure celery juice doesn't taste very nice. At the same time, it doesn't sound very reasonable to live on pure celery juice alone or experiment with unproven and unrealistic celery juice cleanses pushed by mainstream marketing, celebrities and hype gurus.

However, when done right, celery and celery juice can really help you take your health to the next level. This is why this book takes a different approach than most strict celery cleanse books out there.

It shows you how to incorporate celery into healthy and balanced, super low sugar and low carb juicing recipes to help you create optimal health. Without crazy cleanses. Without forcing yourself to drink juices that make you sick. Instead, you can enjoy all the benefits of celery in delicious, tasty and beautiful juices.

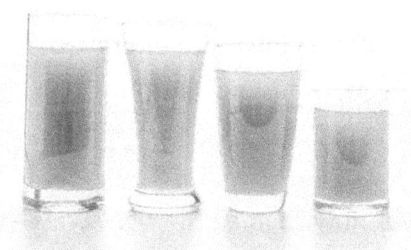

***Celery Juice Recipes That Don't Taste Gross*** **are:**

-low sugar and low carb (compatible with weight loss and low sugar diets)

-combine the healthiest low sugar fruits, veggies, superfoods, and herbs to help you create BALANCE

-taste delicious


**This book is perfect if you want to:**

-enjoy more energy, naturally

-give your body the nutrients it needs to stimulate healing

-speed up massive weight loss, naturally

-improve your health with easy to follow recipes

-have healthy-looking, glowing skin, strong nails, and shiny hair


Whether your goal is to lose weight, enjoy more energy, or learn a few delicious celery juice recipes- you have come to the right place.

With this book, you will discover how to juice the right way – the balanced way, so that you can enjoy all the benefits of celery juice as well as other amazing superfoods.

In this book, the Celery is not playing solo…There is a whole team of amazing superfoods to make celery juice taste amazing so that you can enjoy more variety. You will never get bored with your juices.

The recipes contained in this book, are designed to help you:

-Eliminate sugar cravings.

-Start losing weight naturally.

-Enjoy more energy and vibrant health.

-Help your body heal naturally by giving it a myriad of nutrients to help it get back in balance it deserves.

This guide is NOT designed as a juice fast.

We recommend you follow a balanced, clean food diet with enough calories to meet your nutritional needs (you can check out the first book in the series called **Alkaline Ketogenic Mix** to learn delicious clean food, alkaline keto recipes you will never get bored with).

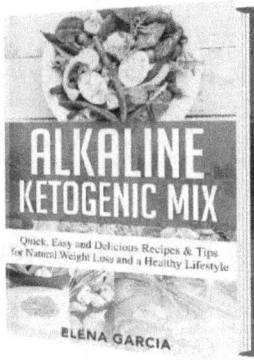

Then, treat juicing, in this case celery juicing as an additional wellness tool.

**Celery is a Simple Superfood...**

Most people think that healthy superfoods are super expensive, hard to pronounce, hard to find and totally unheard of.

Well, it doesn't have to be that way. There are many simple, common-sense superfoods that are easy to find (in your local grocery store) and can help you take your health to the next level.

**The Benefits of Celery**

Celery is very rich in:

-vitamin K (essential vitamin that is needed by the body for blood clotting and other important processes)

-vitamin A (healthy immune system, anti-age, and good vision)

-vitamins B-2 and B-6 (better nutrient absorption)

-vitamin C (healthy immune system and sustainable all-day energy)

Plus, it is also rich in:

-folate

-potassium

-manganese

-pantothenic acid

-dietary fiber

Celery is also low in calories and sugar, making it a perfect choice for a quick and healthy snack (I love snacking on celery sticks with some hummus or guacamole).

It's also an excellent juicing ingredient. When juicing, you give your digestive system a rest, and the nutrients absorb much quicker (and easier), because there is no fiber.

Juicing celery doesn't have to be boring. It can be exciting and fun!

Without any further ado, let's dive right into the food lists...

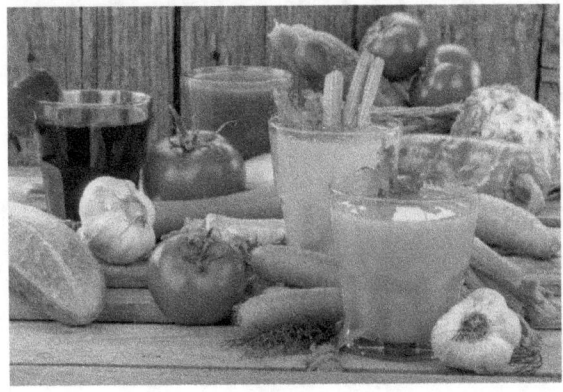

# Juicing Recipes- Food Lists

(aside from our main hero, Celery)

## Recommended Fruit

For healthy juicing, we encourage you to stay away from sugar, including fruit that is high in sugar.

However, low-sugar fruits are allowed, and they will make your celery juice recipes taste great.

**Low Sugar Fruit:**
- Lime
- Lemon
- Grapefruit
- Tomato (yea, it's a fruit)

- Pomegranate

**Other Fruit (in moderation)**

- Orange
- Apple
- Peach
- Pineapple
- Pear

## Recommended Greens to Use in Your Juicing Recipes

- Spinach
- Kale
- Microgreens
- Swiss Chard
- Arugula
- Endive
- Romaine Lettuce
- (and of course, our main hero – Celery!)

+ other fresh leafy greens and greens as well as:

- Parsley
- Mint
- Cilantro

I prefer fresh greens to green powders...but...whenever I go traveling, or I am really pressed for time, I use a delicious green powder that contains 11 superfoods. 11 in 1!

I also like to add it to my recipes as it makes my juices taste really nice while adding a ton of superfoods at the same time. You can learn more about it and how I use it with my recipes on my website (treat it as an additional recommendation):

www.yourwellnessbooks.com/resources

## Vegetables to Use in Your Juices:

- Red bell pepper
- Green bell pepper
- Yellow bell pepper
- Zucchini
- Broccoli
- Asparagus
- Colliflower
- Garlic
- Cucumbers
- Radishes

## Spices & Herbs for Your Juices

The following herbs and spices will make your juices taste delicious. They are also full of anti-inflammatory properties:

- Cinnamon
- Himalaya Salt
- Curry
- Red Chili Powder
- Cumin
- Nutmeg
- Italian spices
- Oregano
- Rosemary
- Lavender
- Mint
- Chamomile
- Fennel
- Cilantro
- Moringa

## Natural Sweeteners and Supplements (Optional)

Stevia (very helpful if you want to make a sweet juice without using sugar or sugar-containing foods or supplements)

- Green Powders
- Spirulina
- Chlorella
- Matcha
- Moringa Powder
- Maca Powder
- Ashwagandha Powder

Again, these are all optional. However, if you are interested in learning more, please visit our private website where I share more complimentary info with my readers. I have listed my favorite brands, green powders, and other health supplements to help you save your time on research:

www.YourWellnessBooks.com/resources

## Good Fats

**These will help your body in better nutrient absorption:**

- Olive oil (organic, cold-pressed)
- Avocado oil
- Hemp oil
- Flaxseed oil
- Coconut oil
- Sesame oil

(please note, there is no need to purchase all of them, one, or two is enough; my two favorites are coconut oil and olive oil)

## Other:

While these are not the main ingredients, they do work really well for some recipes. For example, some juicing recipes may taste way too intense, and so it makes sense to mix them with some healthy nut milk. For example, coconut or cashew milk can make your celery juice recipes taste naturally sweet and creamy.

- Almond milk
- Coconut milk
- Hazelnut milk
- Coconut water
- Herbal infusions
- Organic Apple Cider Vinegar

+ coffee and caffeine, in moderation (for example, you can combine your juice with a little bit of green tea or red tea to get you going in the morning!)

## About the Recipes-Measurements Used in the Recipes

The cup measurement I use is the American Cup measurement.

I also use it for dry ingredients. If you are new to it, let me help you:

If you don't have American Cup measures, just use a metric or imperial liquid measuring jug and fill your jug with your ingredient to the corresponding level. Here's how to go about it:

*1 American Cup= 250ml= 8 Fl.oz.*

For example:
If a recipe calls for 1 cup of almonds, simply place your almonds into your measuring jug until it reaches the 250 ml/8oz marks.

I hope you found it helpful. I know that different countries use different measurements, and I wanted to make things simple for you. I have also noticed that very often those who are used to American Cup measurements complain about metric measurements and vice versa. However, if you apply what I have just explained, you will find it easy to use both.

# Celery Juice Recipes to Help You Thrive!

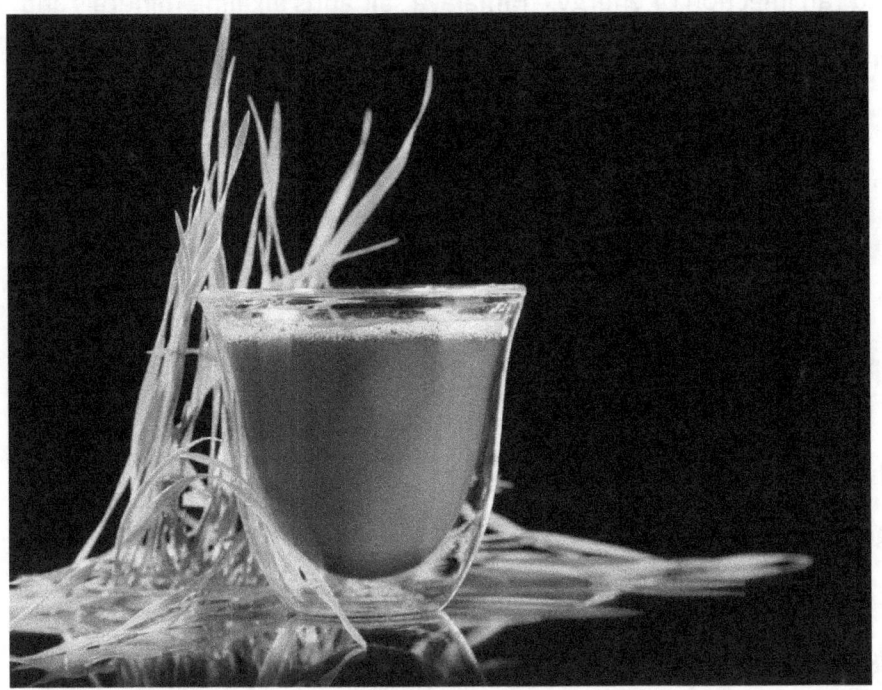

## Recipe#1 Avocado Oil Celery Juice for Energy & Weight Loss

Avocado oil offers good fat to help you absorb the minerals and vitamins from the juice. I love this juice whenever I need "an injection of energy." Himalaya salt adds alkaline minerals and makes this juice taste amazing. If you like spicy juices, feel free to add in some hot sauce, or chili powder.

**Servings: 2**

**Ingredients:**

- 1 lemon, peeled
- 1 lime, peeled
- 6 celery stalks, chopped
- a handful of arugula leaves
- 2 big cucumbers, peeled and chopped
- 2 tablespoons avocado oil
- Himalayan salt to taste
- Optional: hot habanero sauce or chili powder

**Instructions:**

1. Place through a juicer.
2. Juice and combine with the avocado oil and Himalayan salt.
3. Serve in a glass and enjoy!

## Recipe#2 Quit Sugar Cravings Juice

This celery juice recipe is beginner friendly, and it's also designed to help you fight sugar cravings.

The creamy consistency of this juice, micronutrients from green juice and super healthy fats from coconut oil will help you say no to sugar.

**Serves: 2**

**Ingredients:**

- Half cup celery leaves
- 2-inch ginger, peeled
- 2 tablespoons melted coconut oil
- 1 cup of thick coconut milk
- Half teaspoon Ashwagandha
- Optional: stevia to sweeten

**Instructions:**

1. Place the celery and ginger through a juicer.
2. Extract the juice, pour it in a big glass.
3. Combine with coconut milk and oil.
4. Add in the Ashwagandha.
5. Stir well and enjoy.

## Recipe#3 Celery Juice Glow

This recipe uses turmeric that is very alkalizing and also offers anti-inflammatory benefits. When peeling, cutting and juicing turmeric, I recommend you use gloves (unless you want to walk around with orange nails and hands for the next 2 days lol).

**Servings: 2**

**Ingredients:**

- 2 big red bell peppers, chopped
- Half cup celery leaves
- 2 inches of turmeric, peeled (use gloves)
- Half lemon
- 2 tablespoons flax seed oil

**Instructions:**

1. Juice all the ingredients using a juicer.
2. Add in the flax seed oil.
3. Serve in a glass.
4. Enjoy!

## Recipe#4 Celery Immune Tonic

This recipe helps maintain a healthy immune system while helping you enjoy more energy (thanks to Vitamin C).

**Servings: 2**

**Ingredients:**

- half cup celery leaves
- 1 orange, peeled and chopped
- 1 inch of ginger, peeled
- 1 cup of water
- Optional: stevia to sweeten

**Instructions:**

1. Place all the ingredients in a juicer. Juice.
2. Mix with water.
3. Serve chilled with some ice cubes.
4. Enjoy!

## Recipe#5 Super Hydrating Weight Loss Juice

This simple recipe is another easy to follow option for those who don't enjoy drinking pure celery juice. Cucumbers taste really delicious in juices and combine really well with coconut oil and milk.

**Servings: 2**

**Ingredients:**

- 4 big cucumbers, peeled and chopped
- 4 big carrots
- 5 celery sticks
- 2 tablespoons coconut oil, melted
- Himalaya salt to taste, if needed
- Half cup thick coconut milk

**Instructions:**

1. Place all the ingredients through a juicer.
2. Extract the juice.
3. Pour into a chilled glass.
4. Add in the coconut oil and coconut milk.
5. Taste with Himalaya salt if needed.
6. Enjoy!

## Recipe#6 Holistic Balance Celery Juice

Celery offers anti-inflammatory properties and Vitamin C to help you enjoy more energy and take care of your immune system.

Maca powder is a fantastic hormone balancer, and I love using it with this juice. Red bell pepper makes it taste really delicious, and so does the cinnamon and nutmeg powder.

**Servings: 2**

**Ingredients:**

- 1 cup celery, chopped
- 1 inch of ginger, peeled
- 1 red bell pepper
- 2 tablespoons avocado oil
- half teaspoon cinnamon powder
- half teaspoon maca powder
- cinnamon and nutmeg powder to taste

**Instructions:**

1. Juice all the ingredients using a juicer.
2. Pour in a glass.
3. Add in the avocado oil, maca, cinnamon, and nutmeg powder.
4. Stir well, serve and enjoy!

## Recipe#7 On the Go Celery Juice Shot (Liver Lover)

This simple recipe helps detoxify the liver and it works really well first thing in the morning.

**Serves: 1**

**Ingredients:**

- 1 grapefruit
- Half cup celery leaves
- 1 tablespoon avocado oil or coconut oil
- Half cup coconut milk
- Stevia to sweeten, if needed

**Instructions:**

1. Juice grapefruit and celery.
2. In a small glass, combine the juice with the rest of the ingredients.
3. Stir well, drink, and enjoy!
4. To your health!

## Recipe#8 Easy Energy Reboot Juice

This recipe uses coconut water to help you spice up your celery juice and make it taste amazing.

**Serves: 1-2**

**Ingredients:**

- 1 cup of coconut water
- 1 cup celery leaves
- 1-inch ginger
- 1 grapefruit, peeled
- Ice cubes

**Instructions:**

1. Juice the celery, ginger, and grapefruit.
2. Combine with coconut water and ice cubes.
3. Serve and enjoy!

## Recipe#9 Aroma Detox Mix

Cabbage is an excellent source of sulfur, which helps purify the blood and detoxify the liver. Fennel and mint help create a nice flavor while adding in more healing nutrients to help you thrive.

**Servings: 2**

**Ingredients:**

- 1 small red cabbage
- 1 fennel bulb
- A handful of mint leaves
- A handful of celery leaves
- Half cup almond milk (or cashew milk)
- 2 tablespoons melted coconut oil
- Optional- stevia to sweeten

**Procedure:**

1. Juice all the ingredients.
2. Add the almond milk and coconut oil.
3. Stir well.
4. Enjoy!

## Recipe#10 Vitamin C Celery Juice for Natural Energy & Weight Loss

This simple juice recipe offers a fantastic combination of greens with healthy, low sugar fruits and healthy fats. It will help you feel energized while eliminating sugar cravings.

Servings: 1-2

Ingredients:

- 2 grapefruits, peeled
- Half cup celery leaves
- 1-inch ginger
- Half cup coconut milk
- 2 tablespoon flax seed oil or sesame oil
- Optional: stevia to sweeten

Instructions:

1. Juice all the ingredients.
2. Combine with flax seed oil (or sesame oil).
3. If needed, sweeten with stevia.
4. Serve and enjoy!

## Recipe#11 Light Alkaline Keto Juice

This juice is particularly useful for healthy eyesight and beautiful skin as it is packed with Vitamins A and C.

It also helps fight inflammation and takes care of your liver.

**Ingredients:**

- 1 cup radish, cut into smaller pieces
- 5 celery stalks, chopped
- 1-inch ginger
- half lime, peeled
- 1 cup coconut milk
- 1 tablespoon sesame or flax seed oil
- Pinch of Himalayan salt

**Instructions:**

1. Juice the radish, ginger, lime, and fennel.
2. Pour into a glass.
3. Add in the Himalayan salt and oil.
4. Stir in the coconut milk.
5. Stir well, serve and enjoy!

## Recipe#12 Apple Cider Antioxidant Juice for Optimal Energy

This recipe is full of miraculous nutrients to help you get rid of toxins. Its therapeutic properties are enhanced by Apple Cider Vinegar.

Servings: 1-2

Ingredients:

- 2 cucumbers, peeled and sliced
- Half cup of celery leaves
- Half cup of mint leaves
- 2 tablespoons of olive oil
- 1 tablespoon apple cider vinegar (organic)
- Himalayan salt to taste (optional)

Instructions:

1. Juice all the ingredients.
2. Add in the olive oil, apple cider vinegar, Himalayan salt, and black pepper.
3. Serve and enjoy!

***To learn more about Apple Cider Vinegar (for health, home, and beauty), I highly recommend you read my book:

*Apple Cider Vinegar: The Miraculous Natural Remedy!: Holistic Solutions & Proven Healing Recipes for Health, Beauty, and Home*

If your goal is weight loss and body detoxification, you can start adding about 1-2 tablespoons (a day) of quality, organic, apple cider vinegar to your alkaline-keto drinks.

Apple cider vinegar goes really well with therapeutic alkaline keto juices (and also smoothies). It's inexpensive and very effective.

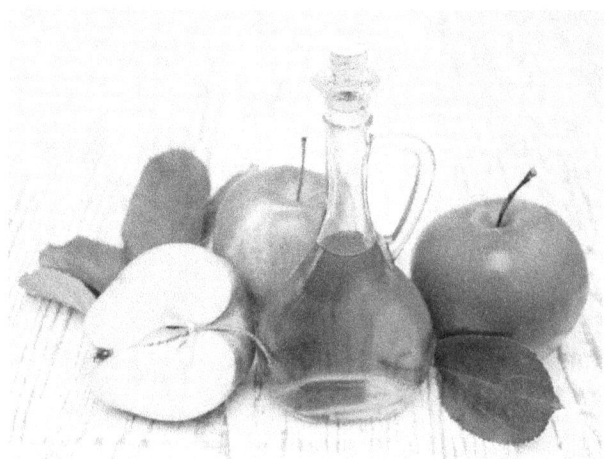

## Recipe#13 Herbal Weight Loss Juice

This recipe fuses the low sugar alkaline fruits with horsetail infusion. Horsetail infusion is an excellent natural remedy to get rid of water retention, lose weight, and burn fat. It's full of alkaline minerals and blends really well with this juice.

**Ingredients:**

- A handful of fresh mint leaves
- A handful of celery leaves
- 1 grapefruit, cut into smaller pieces
- A green apple, cut into smaller pieces
- 1 lime, peeled
- Half inch ginger, peeled
- 1 cucumber, peeled and cut into smaller pieces
- Half cup horsetail infusion cooled down
- Optional: stevia to sweeten

**Instructions:**

1. First, juice all the ingredients.
2. Pour into a glass.
3. Combine with horsetail infusion. Add stevia if needed.
4. Serve and enjoy!

## Recipe#14 Sleep Well Celery Juice

This delicious herbal juice uses verbena- a herb used to stimulate relaxation and peace of mind.

**Servings: 1-2**

**Ingredients:**

- 1 cup verbena infusion, cooled down a bit (use 1 teabag per cup)
- 2 grapefruits, peeled and sliced
- 1 apple, peeled and sliced
- A handful of chopped celery
- A handful of fresh mint leaves
- Stevia to sweeten

**Procedure:**

1. Juice the grapefruits, celery, and mint leaves.
2. Mix the juice with the infusion.
3. Stir well and add stevia for naturally sweet taste.
4. Enjoy!

*Verbena is a pretty safe herb, but there is not enough information to confirm whether it can be used during pregnancy or breastfeeding. The same applies to possible contraindications with other medications. I always recommend consulting with your doctor first.*

## Recipe#15 Pomegranate Celery Anti-Sugar Cravings Juice

This recipe will help you get rid of sugar cravings while feeding your body with a myriad of nutrients it needs to thrive. Pomegranate juice is full of alkaline minerals as well as Vitamin C. It's a natural antioxidant and anti-inflammatory. It blends really well with ginger, turmeric, and celery.

**Servings: 2**

**Ingredients:**

- 1 cup pomegranate seeds
- 1-inch ginger root, peeled
- 1-inch turmeric root, peeled
- A handful of celery leaves
- 2 tablespoons of avocado oil
- Stevia to sweeten (optional)

**Procedure:**

1. Juice the pomegranate seeds, ginger, turmeric, and celery.
2. Pour into a glass.
3. Combine with avocado oil.
4. Stir well.
5. Serve and enjoy!

## Recipe#16 Alkalizing Mojito Juice

It's time for a simple and super healthy, non-alcoholic version of mojito!

**Servings: 2-3**

**Ingredients:**

- 1 cucumber, peeled and sliced
- Half cup fresh mint leaves
- Half cup celery leaves
- 2 limes, peeled and sliced
- A few mint leaves to garnish
- A few lime slices to garnish
- 3 cups alkaline (or filtered) water
- Stevia to sweeten (optional)

**Instructions:**

1. Juice all the ingredients (except the mint and lime slices for garnishing)
2. Pour the fresh juice into a tall water jar or pitcher.
3. Add fresh water and ice cubes.
4. Now, add the mint leaves and lime slices.
5. Stir in well, chill in a fridge for a few hours, and serve.
6. Enjoy!

## Recipe #17 Cucumber Kale and Carrot Juice

While it's hard to eat a mountain of greens and cucumbers, it's easy to drink their juice and get all the vital nutrients in. Avocado oil offers good fat to help you absorb the minerals and vitamins from the juice.

**Servings: 2**

**Ingredients:**

- 2 big carrots, peeled and chopped
- 1 lemon, peeled
- 5 celery stalks, chopped
- A couple dashes of habanero hot sauce
- a handful of kale, chopped
- 2 big cucumbers, peeled and chopped
- a drizzle of avocado oil

**Instructions:**

1. Place through a juicer.
2. Juice.
3. Pour into a glass and add in a couple dashes of habanero hot sauce and avocado oil, if needed.

## Recipe #18 Flavored Celery Juice

While pure celery juice can be a bit hardcore, this recipe is a bit different.

Add in some fresh apples and ginger and you will fall in love with green celery juice.

**Serves: 2**

**Ingredients:**

- 1 cup of celery leaves
- 2 green apples, peeled and chopped
- 2-inch ginger, peeled
- 1 tablespoon melted coconut oil

**Instructions:**

1. Place all the ingredients through a juicer.
2. Extract the juice, pour it in a big glass.
3. Add in some melted coconut oil.
4. Stir well and enjoy.

## Recipe #19 Watermelon Antioxidant Juice

Watermelon, ginger and celery is an excellent combination.

It makes the juice taste nice and helps you get accustomed to juicing celery.

**Servings: 2**

**Ingredients:**

- 1 cup of watermelon, chopped
- 1 cup celery leaves
- 2 inches of ginger, peeled

**Instructions:**

1. Juice all the ingredients using a juicer.
2. Serve in a glass.
3. Enjoy!

## Recipe #20 Simple Apple Lemon Juice

Apples help maintain a healthy digestive system.

Oh, and they make green juices taste great!

**Servings: 2**

**Ingredients:**

- 1 cups of celery leaves
- 2 apples, peeled and chopped
- 1 lemon, peeled and halved
- 1 inch of ginger, peeled
- 1-inch turmeric, peeled

**Instructions:**

1. Place all the ingredients in a juicer.
2. Juice and serve in a glass.
3. Enjoy!

## Recipe #21 Honeydew Melon Green Juice

While a pure green celery juice may be a bit too much for a beginner, adding in some honeydew melon really takes it to a whole new level.

**Servings: 2**

**Ingredients:**

- 4 medium cucumbers, peeled and chopped
- 1 cup of honeydew melon
- 1 cup celery leaves

**Instructions:**

1. Place all the ingredients through a juicer.
2. Extract the juice.
3. Pour into a chilled glass and enjoy!

## Recipe #22 Easy Celery Juice

Red bell peppers are one of my favorite veggies to juice.

They are natural sweet and full of vitamins and minerals. They make any green juice taste amazing. Ginger adds to anti-inflammatory properties.

**Servings: 2**

**Ingredients:**

- 1 cup celery, chopped
- 3 red bell peppers, chopped
- 1 inch of ginger, peeled
- 2 slices of lime, to garnish
- Fresh ice cubes

**Instructions:**

1. Juice all the ingredients using a juicer.
2. Pour in a glass, add in some ice cubes.
3. Garnish with lime slices.
4. Serve and enjoy!

## Recipe #23 Coconut Celery Concoction

Compared to other juicing recipes, this one is relatively simple and quick to make as it leverages the coconut water. Just perfect as a quick, energy boosting juice

**Servings: 2**

**Ingredients:**

- 1 cup celery leaves
- 1 green apple, cut into smaller pieces
- 1 cup of coconut water
- 1 teaspoon cinnamon powder

**Instructions:**

1. Juice the celery and apple.
2. Pour into a glass and mix with 1 cup of coconut water.
3. Stir well, add in 1 teaspoon of cinnamon powder and stir again.

*Green Juice Recipes That Don't Taste Gross*

## Recipe #24 Broccoli and Orange Juice

This juice is great for boosting your energy and stimulating weight loss.

It combines the healing and immune system boosting benefits of Vitamin C from oranges with the detoxifying properties of chlorophyll from the celery.

**Servings: 2**

**Ingredients:**

- 1 cup celery leaves
- 2 oranges, peeled and cut into smaller pieces
- 1 lemon, peeled and cut into smaller pieces
- 1-½ cups of alkaline water

**Instructions:**

1. Place through a juicer.
2. Juice, and pour into a jar or a big glass and add in some water (you can skip this step if you like the intense taste of this juice)
3. Enjoy!

*Green Juice Recipes That Don't Taste Gross*

## Recipe #25 Green Tea High Energy Juice

This uses green tea to help you boost your energy levels and burn fat. Ginger adds to anti-inflammatory properties.

**Servings: 2**

**Ingredients:**

- 2 oranges, peeled and cut into smaller pieces
- 1 green apple, cut to smaller pieces
- Half cup celery leaves
- 1-inch ginger, peeled
- 1 cup green tea, cooled down

**Instructions:**

1. Juice the oranges, ginger and spinach.
2. Pour into a glass or a jar and add in some green tea.
3. Enjoy!

## Recipe #26 A Beta Carotene Powerhouse

This juice is a fantastic combination of oranges, turmeric and carrots to help you have beautiful and healthy-looking skin while enjoying more energy without having to rely on caffeine.

**Servings: 2**

**Ingredients:**

- 6 carrots, peeled and chopped
- 2 oranges, peeled and cut into smaller pieces
- Half cup celery leaves
- 1 lemon, peeled and cut into smaller pieces
- 1 zucchini, peeled and cut into smaller pieces
- 2-inch turmeric, peeled
- A few ice cubes (optional)
- A dash of cinnamon powder (optional)

**Instructions:**

1. Juice all the ingredients.
2. Pour into a glass and add in some ice cubes and a dash of cinnamon powder.
3. Enjoy!

## Recipe #27 A Restorative Antioxidant Juice

This juice is full of antioxidants and beta-carotene to help you have beautiful skin.

**Servings: 2**

**Ingredients:**

- 4 large carrots, peeled and chopped
- 4 tomatoes, cut into smaller pieces
- 6 celery sticks, chopped
- 1 garlic clove, peeled
- 1-inch ginger, peeled

**Instructions:**

1. Juice all the ingredients.
2. Pour into a glass and enjoy!

## Recipe #28 Veggie Medley Juice

Enjoy the wonderful mixture full of ingredients that make you healthy. They also contain antioxidant and elements that will help your body to fight against diseases and help in weight loss.

**Servings: 4**

**Ingredients:**

- 6 medium carrots, peeled and cut into smaller pieces
- 1 beet peeled and cut into smaller pieces
- 3 large tomatoes, cut into smaller pieces
- 1 red bell pepper, chopped
- 4 large celery stalks, chopped

**Instructions:**

1. Juice all the ingredients.
2. Pour into a glass.
3. If needed, season with some Himalaya salt.
4. Enjoy!

## Recipe #29 Coconut Flavored Antioxidant Juice

This recipe has plenty of antioxidants and is full of refreshing nutrients.

While pure green celery juice might be a bit too "hardcore" even for experienced juicing fanatics, it tastes amazing when mixed with other ingredients.

**Servings: 1**

**Ingredients:**

- Half cup celery leaves
- Half cup coconut water or coconut milk
- 2 green apples, chopped

**Instructions:**

1. Juice all the ingredients.
2. Pour into a glass and mix with some coconut water.
3. Enjoy!

## Recipe #30 Mixed Green Juice

This recipe is great if you happen to have some arugula leaves leftovers and don't feel like going for another salad. And yes, arugula juice tastes amazing when mixed with other ingredients!

**Servings: 2**

**Ingredients:**

- 1 cup arugula leaves
- A few pineapples slices
- 4 celery sticks, chopped
- 1 orange, peeled and cut into smaller pieces
- 1 green apple, peeled and cut into smaller pieces

**Instructions:**

1. Place though a juicer.
2. Juice and pour into a glass or a small jar.
3. Enjoy!

## Recipe #31 Tantalizing Green Juice

Once again, we are juicing arugula leaves while adding in some sweetness and vitamin C from Kiwis and anti-inflammatory benefits of ginger. Apple helps in digestion and lime adds even more of vitamin C and refreshing aroma.

**Servings: 2**

**Ingredients:**

- 1 cup arugula leaves
- Half cup celery leaves
- 2 kiwis, peeled
- 1 green apple, cut into smaller pieces
- 1 lime, peeled and cut into smaller pieces
- 1-inch ginger, peeled

**Instructions:**

1. Place all the ingredients though a juicer.
2. Juice and enjoy!

## Recipe #32 Healing Carrot Juice

Carrot juice tastes amazing and when combined with cucumber juice, it will help you stay hydrated and reduce unwanted sugar cravings for hours. Ashwagandha powder is optional here.

But it's a great choice to help you re-balance your energy levels while feeling more relaxed.

**Servings: 2**

**Ingredients:**

- 6 carrots, peeled and chopped
- 3 big cucumbers, peeled and chopped
- Half cup celery leaves
- ¼ teaspoon Ashwagandha powder

**Instructions:**

1. Juice all the ingredients.
2. Pour into a glass and enjoy!

## Recipe #33 Cucumber's Delight

Cucumber contains water that provides a good environment for hydration and therefore contributes to weight loss. Parsley leaves add in a ton of vitamins and nutrients such as Vitamin A, Vitamin C and Iron. Mint helps in digestion and brings an amazing aroma to the table.

**Servings: 2**

**Ingredients:**

- 2 large cucumbers, peeled and chopped
- A handful of fresh mint leaves
- A handful of fresh parsley leaves
- A handful of fresh celery leaves
- Half cup coconut or cashew milk

**Instructions:**

1. Juice all the ingredients.
2. Pour into a glass or a small jar and mix with coconut or cashew milk.
3. Enjoy!

## Recipe #34 Turmeric Celery Juice

Turmeric is full of polyphenols that help well in weight loss.

It's a great addition to your juices and creates a nice, spicy aroma that is very easy to get hooked on.

**Servings: 2**

**Ingredients:**

- 2-inch turmeric, peeled
- 2-inch ginger, peeled
- 4 celery stalks, chopped
- 2 oranges, peeled and cut into smaller pieces
- 1 lemon, peeled and cut into smaller pieces
- Half cup water, filtered

**Instructions:**

1. Juice all the ingredients.
2. Pour into a glass and mix with water.
3. Enjoy!

## Recipe #35 Pineapple Lime Mint Juice

This recipe balances the energy and weight loss stimulating benefits of greens with the sweetness of pineapple.

**Servings: 3-4**

**Ingredients:**

- half cup celery, chopped
- half cup pineapple, chopped
- half cup mint leaves, fresh
- 2 limes, peeled and chopped

**Instructions:**

1. Place through a juicer.
2. Juice and pour into a glass.
3. Enjoy!

## Recipe #36 Antioxidant Nutrition Juice

With orange pomegranate, you are sure of enjoying juice that is full of antioxidants and nutrients that are good for weight loss.

**Servings: 2**

**Ingredients:**

- 1 cup pomegranate seeds
- 1 cup of celery leaves
- 2 oranges, peeled and cut into smaller pieces

**Instructions:**

1. Place through a juicer.
2. Pour into a glass and enjoy!

## Recipe #37 Coconut Flavored Green Juice

The ingredients are rich in phytonutrients and antioxidants. The juice relaxes the body and makes it easy to lose extra pounds.

**Servings: 2**

**Ingredients:**

- 1 cup celery leaves
- 2 tablespoons avocado oil
- 1 cup pineapple, chopped
- 1 green apple, chopped

**Instructions:**

1. Place all the ingredients through a juicer.
2. Juice and pour into a glass
3. Enjoy!

## Recipe#38 Creamy, Anti-Inflammatory Breakfast Delight

Yes, this juice is great as a natural drink. It is packed with nutrients, and uses an army of anti-inflammatory spices.

**Servings: 1-2**

**Ingredients:**

- 2 beets, peeled
- 1 red apple, peeled
- 2 red bell peppers
- 1 cup celery leaves
- 1-inch ginger, peeled
- 1 cup coconut milk or coconut cream (natural, organic)
- 2 tablespoons of coconut oil
- 2 tablespoons of chia seeds
- Stevia to sweeten (optional)
- Half teaspoon cinnamon powder
- Half teaspoon nutmeg powder

**Instructions:**

1. Wash and chop the veggies.
2. Juice and add some ginger too.
3. Mix the fresh juice with coconut milk (or coconut cream, just be sure to choose coconut milk that has a thick consistency).
4. Add the cinnamon and nutmeg powder. Sweeten with stevia. Stir well.
5. Place 2 tablespoons of chia seeds on top.

## Recipe#39 Get Energized Antioxidant Juice

I don't know about you, but I love combining my juices with teas and herbal infusions. Especially green tea!

Perfect recipe to help you stay energized for hours, without getting overstimulated.

**Servings: 1-2**

**Ingredients:**

- 1 cup of green tea, cooled down
- 2 oranges
- A handful of celery leaves
- Optional: stevia to sweeten if needed

**Instructions:**

1. Juice the celery and oranges.
2. Combine with green tea, serve and enjoy!

## Recipe#40 Green Balance Party Juice

Fennel bulb is naturally sweet and can be an amazing addition to your celery juices. It is also rich in potassium, vitamin A, calcium, iron, vitamin B6, magnesium, as well as phosphorus, zinc, copper, selenium, beta-carotene and manganese.

**Servings: 2**

**Ingredients:**

- 4 big cucumbers, peeled
- Half cup celery leaves
- Half fennel bulb
- 1-inch ginger, peeled
- 1 big, ripe pear to taste
- Half cup water, filtered, preferably alkaline

**Instructions:**

1. Wash and chop all the veggies.
2. Peel the cucumber, lemon and ginger.
3. Place through a juicer.
4. Add some water.
5. Stir well, drink and enjoy!

## Recipe#41 Delicious Creamy Beet Juice

**Beets are rich in** antioxidant and anti-inflammatory phytonutrients, like betalains. Moreover, beetroot is also a diuretic, helping fight water retention, edema, and cellulite.

Servings: 2-3

Ingredients:

- half cup celery leaves
- 2 beets (with the leaves if possible)
- 1 apple, peeled
- 2 carrots, peeled, unless organic
- 2 limes, peeled
- half teaspoon powdered cinnamon
- half cup coconut milk

Instructions:

1. Juice all the ingredients.
2. Now, stir in the cinnamon powder.
3. Mix with coconut milk, serve and enjoy!

## Recipe#42 Spicy Green Celery Juice

This juice can be a fantastic, natural remedy for colds and flu.

**Servings: 1-2**

**Ingredients:**

- Half inch turmeric root, peeled
- Half inch ginger root, peeled
- 1 red bell pepper
- half cup celery leaves
- 1 big tomato
- 1 lime, peeled

**Instructions:**

1. Wash and chop all the ingredients.
2. Juice and enjoy!

## Recipe #43 Gazpacho Celery Juice

This recipe tastes a bit like Spanish gazpacho and can get you hooked on celery…

**Serves: 1**

**Ingredients:**

- 2 big tomatoes
- 2 big cucumbers, peeled
- 4 celery sticks, chopped
- 1 tablespoon olive oil
- Himalayan salt and black pepper to taste

**Instructions:**

1. Juice all the ingredients.
2. Add in olive oil, Himalayan salt and black pepper.
3. Stir well, serve and enjoy!

## Recipe #44 "Replenish Yourself" Juice

Coconut water can be a great addition to your celery juicing recipes. It's excellent for optimal hydration and it contains many natural minerals, such as Magnesium.

**Serves: 2-3**

**Ingredients:**

- 1 cup coconut water
- 2-inch ginger
- 1 garlic clove, peeled
- 2 grapefruits
- 1 cup celery leaves

**Instructions:**

1. Juice all the ingredients.
2. Combine with coconut water and ice cubes.
3. Serve and enjoy!

## Recipe #45 "Red Pepper Detox" Juice

Fennel and mint help create a sweet flavor while contributing more healing nutrients to help you thrive.

**Servings: 2**

**Ingredients:**

- 2 big red bell peppers
- 1 fennel bulb
- A handful of mint leaves (optional)
- 1 cup celery leaves
- Half cup of coconut milk
- 1 tablespoon avocado oil
- Optional- stevia to sweeten

**Instructions:**

1. Juice all the ingredients.
2. Add the coconut milk and avocado oil.
3. Stir well, adding stevia if needed.
4. Enjoy!

## Recipe #46 "Liver Lover" Juice

Grapefruits are very rich in phytonutrients called limonoids that promote the production of antioxidant enzymes. These help the liver to remove toxic compounds easier, thereby protecting the liver in the process.

**Servings: 2**

**Ingredients:**

- 2 grapefruits, peeled
- Half cup celery leaves
- 1 inch of fresh root ginger, peeled
- Half cup water, filtered, preferably alkaline
- 2 tablespoons of Udo's Choice (you can also use cold-pressed flax oil)
- Pinch of Himalayan salt
- 1 tablespoon of avocado or olive oil

**Instructions:**

1. Juice all the ingredients.
2. Add the water, Udo's Choice, Himalayan salt and olive or avocado oil.
3. Stir well and drink to your health.

## Recipe #47 Creamy Chia Juice

What I really like about this recipe is its natural creaminess thanks to cashew milk and chia seeds.

**Servings: 2-3**

**Ingredients:**

- 2 cucumbers, peeled
- 1-inch ginger, peeled
- Half cup celery leaves
- 1 tablespoon avocado oil or olive oil
- 1 cup of raw cashew milk (unsweetened)
- Pinch of black pepper and Himalayan salt if needed

**Instructions:**

1. Juice the cucumbers, ginger and celery.
2. Pour into a glass.
3. Stir in some olive or avocado oil and mix in the cashew milk while adding black pepper and Himalayan salt.
4. Drink immediately.
5. Enjoy the energy!

# Part 3- Book 3

# Paleo Drinks

*Delicious and Easy Paleo Drink Recipes for Natural Weight Loss and A Healthy Lifestyle*

By Elena Garcia

Copyright Elena Garcia © 2019

All rights reserved. No part of this publication may be reproduced, stored in a retrieval system, or transmitted, in any form or by any means, electronic, mechanical, photocopying, recording or otherwise, without the prior written permission of the author and the publishers.

The scanning, uploading, and distribution of this book via the Internet or via any other means without the permission of the author is illegal and punishable by law. Please purchase only authorized electronic editions, and do not participate in or encourage electronic piracy of copyrighted materials.

**Disclaimer**

A physician has not written the information in this book. It is advisable that you visit a qualified dietician so that you can obtain a highly personalized treatment for your case, especially if you want to lose weight effectively. This book is for informational and educational purposes only and is not intended for medical purposes. Please consult your physician before making any drastic changes to your diet.

All information in this book has been carefully researched and checked for factual accuracy. However, the author and publishers make no warranty, expressed or implied, that the information contained herein is appropriate for every individual, situation or purpose, and assume no responsibility for errors or omission. The reader assumes the risk and full responsibility for all actions and the author will not be held liable for any loss or damage, whether consequential, incidental, and special or otherwise, that may result from the information presented in this publication.

The book is not intended to provide medical advice or to take the place of medical advice and treatment from your personal physician. Readers are advised to consult their own doctors or other qualified health professionals regarding the treatment of medical conditions. The author shall not be held liable or responsible for any misunderstanding or misuse of the information contained in this book. The information is not intended to diagnose, treat or cure any disease.

# Introduction

Thank You for purchasing this book. It means you are very serious about your health and wellbeing. Whether your goal it to lose weight, enjoy more energy or learn a few delicious healing recipes- you have come to the right place.

You are probably thinking...what? Paleo Drinks? What kind of a recipe book am I getting myself into? Does it mean I will be making some meat smoothies or juicing bacon? How about some egg tea?

The answer is no. This book will help you enrich your diet with a myriad of natural super healthy detoxifying drinks that will make you look and feel amazing. You will get a practical understanding of the best paleo drink recipes that are full of vitamins and minerals so that you can enjoy unstoppable energy.

The truth is, most people don't focus enough on what they drink. And they skip this amazing opportunity of vibrant health through paleo friendly hydration.

In case you are new to the paleo diet, the following pages will give you the easiest to follow healthy and balanced paleo lifestyle blueprint that is very easy to understand. Then, we will dive into paleo drink recipes as this is what this guide is all about.

So even if you are new to a healthy lifestyle-no worries, we got you covered.

And if you are already enjoying the wellness benefits that transitioning to a paleo diet and life offers, I am sure that the recipes contained in this book, will help you take it to the next level.

My goal is to make it as simple and doable as possible by giving you all the information, inspiration and recipes you need to transform your body while enjoying the process.

So...first of all, what is a paleo diet? Some kind of a cult? Or maybe a fad?
Well, some people in the health community love creating cults around diets, that's for sure.

But we like to keep it as easy to understand and follow as possible. Then, our goal is to make it easy, doable and fun- especially for a busy person.

Eating a paleo diet means- eating foods that can be hunted or gathered while excluding processed foods.

And so, a paleo eater chooses:
- organic meat
- fresh fish and seafood
- organic eggs
- veggies
- fruits
- nuts & seeds
- herbs and spices (yes, they are paleo too!)

There is no dairy on a paleo diet. Instead of butter, it's recommended to use natural oils such as coconut oil or avocado oil. Milk is also off a paleo diet. Luckily, coconut milk and all kinds of nut milks are allowed. We are talking creamy cashew milk, aromatic coconut milk, delicious hazelnut milk. There are so many options out there!

To keep it simple – we just want to eat a natural, balanced diet and get rid of or reduce all processed foods.
Some people go paleo full time. Some do it part time. The truth is, even if you eat this way about 80% of time, you are good to go.

In this day and age, it's hard to keep a perfect diet.

But, creating vibrant health is all about balance, progress and healthy choices.

Most Paleo Diet beginners I talk to, think that going paleo is all about eating lots of meat and that's it. Huge mistake. Our Paleolithic ancestors were also gatherers. So, aside from eating meat, they would also eat veggies, fruits, nuts and seeds. Oh, and herbs…

Nothing is every black and white. Balance is the key. That is how vibrant health is created.
Add to it relaxation, mindfulness, kindness and…some paleo drinks, which is what this recipe book is all about.

You see, even the healthiest paleo diet is doomed to fail if we forget about proper hydration.
Imagine our ancestors…I wonder…did they run on coffee all day? Drinking coffee and eating meat all day.

Does that sound reasonable?
Of course not. And you don't need to be an expert in nutrition to admit that.

I know I am exaggerating here. But, unfortunately, most people rely too much on coffee and forget about other drink alternatives.
That leads to dehydration. When you are dehydrated it's hard to focus, think clearly, feel motivated or even eat healthy.

It's very easy to misinterpret the feeling of dehydration as "I am feeling hungry again".

Now, it's time to re-connect with our Paleolithic ancestors and dive deep into a healthy, balanced lifestyle by giving yourself the optimal hydration we deserve.

That is why I decided to write this book. I want you to dive into my best paleo drink recipes that include smoothies, juices and teas.

It's time to nourish your body with a myriad of nutrients and healing recipes. Most people overlook the simple superfoods, herbs, fruits and veggies that can be turned into natural and paleo friendly concoctions to help you stay energized.

This book is divided into 4 parts. The first part includes delicious paleo smoothies, including both naturally sweet smoothies as well as super tasty veggie smoothies. Many veggie smoothies can be turned into comforting soups, and you can even add in some meat or fish leftovers.

The second part is all about paleo juices, and the third part will help you discover the best of paleo friendly herbs, teas and infusions.

The fourth part is optional as it includes a mini paleo "crash course" to help you understand how this diet works.

Healthy eating is very easy when you commit to becoming resourceful.

And it is my ultimate passion and mission. Through this book, I want to inspire you to start adding more delicious and nutritious paleo drinks to your diet.

To your health,
Enjoy!

## About the Recipes-Measurements Used in the Recipes

The cup measurement I use is the American Cup measurement.

I also use it for dry ingredients. If you are new to it, let me help you:

If you don't have American Cup measures, just use a metric or imperial liquid measuring jug and fill your jug with your ingredient to the corresponding level. Here's how to go about it:

*1 American Cup= 250ml= 8 fl.oz.*

For example:

If a recipe calls for 1 cup of almonds, simply place your almonds into your measuring jug until it reaches the 250 ml/8oz mark.

I hope you found it helpful. I know that different countries use different measurements and I wanted to make things simple for you. I have also noticed that very often those who are used to American Cup measurements complain about metric measurements and vice versa. However, if you apply what I have just explained, you will find it easy to use both.

# Part 1 Paleo Smoothie Recipes

Paleo smoothies are tasty, easy and quick to prepare even on a busy schedule. They can be used as a quick snack or breakfast.

These smoothies are great for weight loss being full of fiber, vitamins and minerals. Some people find them useful for fasting or as a meal replacement.

You can play around with many of the ingredients and come up with your own favorites. You can leave things out or add some new ones so that you create the taste you love. That's what I love about them, they are so changeable but still so tasty and nutritious. Change things up and try something new. Have fun, be creative!

***Note: be sure to wash all the fruits and veggies before turning them into smoothies.***

## Recipe #1 Banana Breakfast

This banana smoothie is perfect for breakfast and incorporates spirulina and kale, helping you to get in some extra nutrients in this morning smoothie. It is an energy boost that will keep you feeling full. You will get fiber, nutrients, and good, paleo friendly carbs in one glass! Spirulina is an excellent superfood supplement to add to many foods or drinks to assist in weight loss.

**Serves 1-2**

**Ingredients:**

- 1 green apple, peeled
- 1 banana, peeled
- 1 tablespoon Spirulina
- ½ cup kale, peeled
- 1 cup coconut milk
- A few ice cubes

**Instructions:**

1. Place all the above ingredients in your blender.
2. Blend well.
3. Serve and enjoy!

## Recipe #2 Berry Blaster

I love coconut water in my smoothie recipes because it is super hydrating and it has a wonderful flavor. When people get dehydrated one of the first signs is the feeling of hunger. So, the good news is- by keeping yourself hydrated you will prevent unhealthy snack cravings.

**Serves: 2**

**Ingredients:**

- 1.5 cup of coconut water
- 1 cup blueberries, 1 cup of blackberries, 1 cup of raspberries (fresh)
- 1.5 cup spinach
- 2 tablespoons raw organic honey
- ¾ cup ice

**Instructions:**

1. Put all ingredients in a blender.
2. Pulse to desired consistency.
3. Enjoy!

## Recipe #3 Paleo Hunger Hunter Smoothie

Avocados are full of healthy fats and nutrients. One half contains six grams of fiber. They contain protein, potassium and many vitamins. They keep my stomach full for hours. They are a super fruit. Not to mention they will add a lot of creaminess to any smoothie.

Egg yolks are a great addition to any smoothie on the paleo plan. Make sure they are organic and free-range or pasture raised. The yolks contain protein and omega 3s. They will fill you up and smash your hunger induced cravings.

**Serves: 1**

**Ingredients:**

- 1 avocado, peeled and pitted
- 1 large banana
- 2 cups of coconut or almond milk
- A cup of ice
- ¾ cup of kale
- ¾ cup of fresh spinach
- 2 egg yolks, organic

**Instructions:**

1. In a blender, add all the above ingredients except for the ice. Blend well.
2. Add ice and pulse until smooth.
3. Enjoy!

## Recipe #4 Veggie Medley

Vegetables are an essential part of weight loss because they contain all of the vitamins our bodies require to run optimally. Unfortunately, most people struggle with putting the veggies together. Not everyone enjoys a big bowl of salad with their meals. That is why paleo smoothies are an amazing solution. You can blend the veggies with some fruits and make sure you easily get all your healthy greens in, without even thinking about it.

**Serves: 2-3**

**Ingredients:**

- 2 handfuls of kale, chopped
- 2 stalks celery, chopped
- 1 cucumber, peeled and chopped
- 1 zucchini, peeled and chopped
- 1 lemon, peeled
- 1 big banana, peeled and chopped
- 2 cups almond milk, or any other paleo nut milk of your choice

**Instructions:**

1. Blend all and pulse in ice.
2. Enjoy!

## Recipe #5 Easy Snack Smoothie

This smoothie will fill you up and you will not feel engorged or weighed down. It's just perfect when you feel like snacking. Why not drink this delicious smoothie instead?

Cranberries are high in vitamin C, among many other antioxidants. They help the body's conversion of glucose to energy.

**Serves: 2**

**Ingredients:**

- 2 teaspoons melted coconut oil
- 2 organic free-range egg yolks
- Handful of spinach
- 1 banana, peeled
- ½ cup cranberries
- 1 cup coconut water
- 1 cup coconut milk

**Instructions:**

1. Blend all and pulse in ice.
2. Enjoy!

## Recipe #6 Healing Energy in a Glass

Feeling fatigued? You don't need another coffee. You already know that too much coffee can make you feel anxious...Try this smoothie instead as it will help you stay energized naturally.

Pepitas/pumpkin seeds are paleo-friendly and are great for weight loss. They contain quite a bit of zinc, which is important because it helps us produce testosterone to burn fat and build muscle. They also have magnesium and iron. Instant energy boost!

**Serves: 3**

**Ingredients:**

- ½ cup broccoli florets, chopped
- 1 cup spinach
- 1 egg yolk
- 1 tablespoon almond butter
- 1 tablespoon coconut oil
- Handful of pepitas
- 1 cucumber, peeled and chopped
- 1 ½ cup coconut water
- A few ice cubes

**Instructions:**

1. Blend all the above ingredients together in a blender except ice.
2. When well blended add the half cup ice and pulse.
3. Enjoy!

## Recipe #7 Mental Energy Smoothie

Blueberries have been shown to improve brain function and motor skills. The recommendation is 1 cup/day. Avocado helps to lower blood pressure and allows for healthy blood flow; both of which affect brain function positively.

This smoothie is perfect if you need to study, work or concentrate for long periods of time.

**Serves: 2**

**Ingredients:**

- 1 cup blueberries, fresh
- 1 avocado, peeled and pitted
- 1 cup of almond or cashew milk
- 1/2 cup baby spinach

**Instructions:**

1. Place all the above ingredients in a blender, mix well and enjoy!

## Recipe #8 Berry Antioxidant Weight Loss Smoothie

Blackberries contain more antioxidants than all of the other fruits on the Paleo plan. They are also rich in fiber content to help you stay full for hours, without feeling hungry.

**Serves: 3-4**

**Ingredients:**
- 1 cup of blueberries, fresh
- 1 cup blackberries, fresh
- 1 cup raspberries, fresh
- 2 cups almond milk
- ½ large banana, peeled
- Handful of greens of your choice

**Instructions:**
1. Blend all.
2. Serve and Enjoy!

## Recipe #9 Mango Green Madness

This simple recipe combines the sweetness of mangos with the healing, alkalizing properties of spinach. Raw honey helps maintain a healthy immune system.

**Serves: 2**

**Ingredients:**

- 1 mango, peeled and sliced
- ½ banana, peeled
- 1 cup spinach
- 1 tablespoon raw honey
- A few ice cubes (optional)

**Instructions:**

1. Add all the above ingredients in a blender and blend well.
2. Pour and enjoy!

## Recipe #10 Sweet Date Healing

This is one smoothie that I turn to whenever I am craving sweets.

The cinnamon in this smoothie helps to regulate blood sugar and insulin levels in the body.

And it tastes so delicious you crave more and more of it.

*Go for it, it's all guilt free.*

**Serves: 1-2**

**Ingredients:**

- 1/3 cup Medjool dates, pitted
- 1/2 cup ice
- 1 cup of almond or any other nut milk of your choice
- ½ avocado (peeled and pitted)
- 1 teaspoon of cinnamon powder
- Optional: 1 teaspoon melted coconut oil

**Instructions:**

1. Place all the above ingredients into the blender and mix/blend well.

## Recipe #11 Vegetable Desire

After I had been eating a healthy, balanced paleo diet for a few months, I craved raw veggies constantly. That is why I came up with this simple veggie smoothie recipe, to make sure I get my daily portions of minerals and vitamins to look and feel amazing.

**Serves: 2**

**Ingredients:**

- 1 cup collard greens, Swiss chard, spinach mix
- 2 celery stalks, chopped
- ½ cup broccoli florets, chopped
- 1 cucumber, peeled and chopped
- 1 handful dandelion greens
- 2 Medjool dates
- 1 cup coconut water
- ½ c. ice

**Instructions:**

1. Place all the listed ingredients except for ice in a blender and mix/blend well.
2. Pulse in some ice.
3. Pour and enjoy.

**Recipe #12 Simple Cream Smoothie**

This is an amazing smoothie recipe if you are craving something sweet and creamy.

**Serves: 1**

**Ingredients:**

- 1 avocado (peeled and pitted)
- 1 small banana, peeled
- 1 tablespoon chia seeds
- 1 teaspoon cinnamon powder
- 1 teaspoon cocoa
- 1 cup coconut milk

**Instructions:**

1. Blend all except the ice for as long as possible.
2. Pulse in ice or skip the ice and freeze for ½ hour.
3. Enjoy!

## Recipe #13 Mango Protein Smoothie

This smoothie is very high in protein and good fats which makes it an excellent breakfast smoothie as it will help you stay full till lunch.

**Serves: 2**

**Ingredients:**

- 1 frozen mango, chopped
- 3 tablespoons-soaked almonds
- 1 tablespoon powdered chia seeds
- 1.5 cup almond milk
- 1 cup spinach
- Half avocado, peeled, pitted
- Handful of blueberries

**Instructions:**

1. Blend all in a blender.
2. Enjoy the fruit of your labor!

## Recipe #14 Guava Smoothie

Ginger and papaya are an amazing digestive mix. We are also getting in some greens to stay energized and guava to make it taste delicious.

**Serves: 2**

**Ingredients:**

- 1/2 cup of guava, chopped
- 1/2 cups spinach
- ½ lemon, peeled
- 1 teaspoon grated ginger
- ½ cup papaya, chopped
- 1 cup coconut water
- Ice, as needed

**Instructions:**

1. Place all the above ingredients in a blender. Carefully mix to attain the desired consistency.
2. Pulse in ice.
3. Enjoy!

## Recipe #15 Cucumber Hydrating Green Smoothie

Cucumber is ultra-refreshing and full of healthy alkaline minerals such as magnesium. Cilantro naturally works as a diuretic for the body.

This smoothie can also be served as a soup (warm or chilled).

If you want to serve it as a soup, I recommend you add in some hard-boiled eggs or smoked salmon. It really tastes delicious.
Enjoy!

**Serves: 1**

**Ingredients:**

- 2 cucumbers, peeled
- 1 celery stalk
- 1 avocado (peeled and pitted)
- Handful of cilantro
- 1 cup filtered water
- Pinch of Himalaya salt
- Pinch of black pepper
- Juice of half a lemon to taste

**Instructions:**

1. Blend all and refresh!

## Recipe #16 Paleo Zucchini Zip

Zucchini is a wonderful option to be considered for the aim of weight loss. It contains few calories and is packed with vitamins and flavonoids. You can eat a ton of it without eating a bunch of calories. While, on its own, it may seem a bit boring, when blended with fruits and spices it really tastes amazing!

**Serves: 1-2**

**Ingredients:**
- 1 zucchini
- ½ green apple
- ¼ teaspoon cinnamon
- 1 cup spinach
- 1 cup coconut water
- ½ cup ice

**Instructions:**
1. Blend all ingredients.
2. Pulse ice and enjoy!

## Recipe #17 Watermelon Dream

Watermelon is one of the most hydrating fruits and is also is an excellent fruit for weight loss. Aside from being low in calories it is packed with nutrients. This recipe is perfect if you are working out. Watermelon is rich in the amino acid called citrulline and is useful in muscle recovery. Drink to your health!

Oh and we are sneaking in some greens too...

**Serves: 2**

**Ingredients:**

- 1 cup chopped watermelon
- 1 cup strawberries (fresh or frozen)
- A few broccoli florets
- ½ cup spinach
- 1 cup coconut water
- 1 teaspoon maca powder
- ½ cup ice (you can omit if using frozen berries)

**Instructions:**

1. Put all in a blender and mix to desired consistency.
2. Enjoy!

## Recipe #18 Mediterranean Gazpacho Smoothness

Gazpacho is a traditional Spanish vegetable smoothie-like soup. It can be served both as a soup as well as a smoothie. It's one of my favorite lunch-time Paleo smoothies.

Not only can it fill your stomach for hours and give you the necessary energy and healthy fats you need (olive oil), but also tastes out of this earth.

If you decide to serve this recipe as a soup, my suggestion is to add in some ham, fried bacon or hard-boiled eggs for protein. You can also add in some chopped veggies of your choice, or any meat leftovers.

Perfect meal for a busy schedule!

**Serves: 2**

**Ingredients:**

- 2 tablespoons green onion, sliced
- 2 tablespoons white ground pepper, chopped
- 2 tablespoon fresh lemon juice
- A handful of chopped celery
- ½ cup cucumber, peeled and chopped
- ¼ cup carrot, peeled and chopped
- 1 ½ cups peeled, diced and seeded tomatoes
- ½ cup almond, dairy free yogurt (you can also use coconut yoghurt)
- Half cup water, filtered
- 1 teaspoon ground black pepper
- 1 tablespoon extra-virgin olive oil

- 1 small clove of garlic
- Himalaya salt to taste
- 8 fresh basil leaves to garnish

**Instructions:**

1. Put all ingredients except basil leaves in blender and mix well.
2. If needed, add some more water and blend again.
3. Allow the gazpacho to cool.
4. Serve chilled in a bowl, decorated with basil leaves. Enjoy!

## Recipe #19 Celery Citrus Snack

This hydrating and refreshing smoothie is one of my favorites for warm weather. It's super hydrating and full of vital nutrients. The mint and citrus twist add an interesting flavor combination to the same vegetables that are used in most Paleo smoothies.

Mint is great for weight loss. Something about the taste suppresses appetite. Throw it in a smoothie and you will have added appetite suppression.

**Serves: 1**

**Ingredients:**
- 2 celery stalks
- 1 small cucumber, peeled and chopped
- Handful of spinach
- ½ lemon peeled
- 1 cup coconut milk
- ½ cup ice
- 3 mint leaves

**Instructions:**
1. Place the above ingredients in your blender and process until smooth.
2. Enjoy!

### Recipe #20 Kale Green Powder Cup

Kale is a fabulous weight loss food because not only is it high in fiber to clean you out and help you feel full, it is packed with phytonutrients, tons of vitamins and minerals.

It is a super food and a sure-fire way to make sure you get a lot of it into your system every day is by supplementing what you eat with what you drink.

**Serves: 1**

**Ingredients:**

- 1 cup kale leaves
- 1 teaspoon spirulina powder
- 1 cup cashew milk (it tastes very creamy, however you can use any other nut milk)
- Half lemon, peeled
- 1 tablespoon coconut oil
- 1 green apple

**Instructions:**

1. Mix all in a blender.
2. Pour into your cup and enjoy!

## Recipe #21 Delicious Baobab Smoothie

Baobab is rich in antioxidants, vitamin C, and potassium as well as digestive enzymes and probiotics. It also optimizes the absorption of iron.

And of course, thanks to fiber, it helps you lose weight, and then keep it off. Tahini makes this smoothie super nutritious - sesame seeds provide the body with valuable nutrients, are a source of protein, magnesium, vitamin B12, healthy fat, calcium required for blood vessels, carbohydrates, amino acids, antioxidants (sesamol and sesamolin) – all this causes human cells to age more slowly. This smoothie is a perfect meal replacement and with its natural protein and healthy fats, it will help you feel full for hours.

**Serves: 1-2**

**Ingredients:**

- ½ teaspoon baobab fruit powder
- ½ teaspoon yacon powder / lucuma
- 1 cup fresh blueberries
- 1 cup almond milk
- Juice of 2 lemons
- 1/3 avocado
- 1 tablespoon of Tahini
- Optional: maple syrup, a few dates or stevia to sweeten, if needed

**Instructions:**

1. Using a blender, mix all the above ingredients together.
2. Enjoy!

## Recipe #22 Choco Power Brain Smoothie

Cocoa has plenty antioxidants like the flavonoids and procyanidins (good agents for anti-ageing). It regenerates the body after exercise, both physically and mentally. It also significantly improves the functioning of the brain and memory.

Personally, I love this smoothie as a healthy, guilt-free treat.
At the same time, it's one of my favorite "power brain" smoothies for long writing sessions.

**Serves: 1-2**

**Ingredients:**

- 1 cup raw almond milk (without sugar)
- 6 pitted Medjool dates
- 1 small banana
- 3 tablespoons organic cocoa powder or few organic, paleo-friendly dark chocolate cubes (70%-90% is the best)
- 1 teaspoon melted coconut oil
- 1 teaspoon maca powder
- 1 teaspoon cinnamon powder
- 1 teaspoon chia seed powder (or chia seeds)

**Instructions:**

1. Put the almond milk, the dates and cocoa/chocolate in a blender first. Mix well. Add the banana, and blend again until everything is perfectly smooth.
2. Serve.
3. You may want to add or subtract from the cocoa, just adjust it to your own taste.
4. Enjoy!

## Recipe #23 The Smashing Pumpkin

Frozen blueberries, ground cloves and fresh ginger will give this smoothie a very fresh, unique and enticing taste. I fell in love with it so many years ago! Pumpkin makes this smoothie full of good carbs that will help you stay energized for hours. You can also serve this smoothie as a thick, cold soup, or add in some nuts and seeds and serve it as a delicious, paleo smoothie bowl.

**Serves: 1**

**Ingredients:**

- 1 cup unsweetened almond or coconut milk
- ½ cup frozen blueberries
- A handful of cashew nuts
- ¼ teaspoon fresh ginger
- a teaspoon of ground cloves
- ½ cup smashed pumpkin

**Instructions:**

1. Put all ingredients in a blender and mix well.
2. Add ginger
3. Enjoy!

## Recipe #24 Greens Sneaker

This smoothie is perfect for people who don't really like the idea of eating green salads. I get that. I know that veggies and greens can get boring.

That is why, this recipe is just perfect, as you can easily get 2 cups of greens without even trying.

**Serves: 2**

**Ingredients:**

- 2 cups kale, fresh
- 2 cups coconut milk
- 1/2 cup pineapple, chopped
- 1 big kiwi, peeled
- 1 lime, peeled
- 1 teaspoon cinnamon powder
- A few fresh dates, pitted

**Instructions:**

1. Place all the other ingredients in a blender.
2. Blend and enjoy with ice cubes.

## Recipe #25 Berry Best

This smoothie is a wonder in itself. It combines natural fiber and vitamin C from fresh fruits with an immune system boosting properties of honey.
To your health!

**Serves: 3**

**Ingredients:**

- 1 cup of coconut water
- 1 cup of blackberry
- 1 cup of raspberry
- 1 teaspoon chlorella powder
- A dash of honey
- Ice cubes

**Instructions:**

1. Blend all the ingredients in a food processor.
2. Pour in a tall glass, chill out the smoothie with ice cubes.

## Recipe #26 Watermelon Berry Dream

Guava with watermelon and berries is a killer combination and it is a treat to Paleo eaters. Other than being super delicious and taste buds friendly, ingredients used in this smoothie also promote weight loss, as guava and watermelon provide the essential amount of fiber and the huge water content in watermelon helps keep the stomach full for a longer time, thereby curbing food cravings.

**Serves: 2-3**

**Ingredients:**

- 1 cup of watermelon, cubed, seeded and chilled
- Half cup strawberries
- Half cup blueberries
- 1.5 cup water, filtered
- ½ cup guava, chopped
- Ice cubes (optional)

**Instructions:**

1. Blend until thoroughly combined and smooth.
2. Toss in some ice cubes and enjoy.

## Recipe #27 Papaya Weight Loss Surprise

Papaya is one of the best fruits to have while trying to reduce weight. It can also effectively help reduce bloating and other digestive problems. It combines really well with coconut oil and cinnamon powder, to help you reduce sugar cravings

**Serves: 1-2**

**Ingredients:**

- 1 small papaya, peeled, seeded and cubed
- 2 big carrots, peeled and chopped
- 1 cup coconut milk
- 1 tablespoon coconut oil
- 1 teaspoon cinnamon powder

**Instructions:**

1. Blend until smooth.
2. Toss in a few ice cubes and serve chilled.
3. Enjoy!

## Recipe #28 Creamy Peach

This creamy smoothie is awesome for hot summer days. It's full of superfoods too. For example, maca powder helps re-balance hormones and Ashwagandha is an ancient Ayurvedic herb that helps sooth anxiety.

To learn more about this herb, I warmly invite you to read by book: "ASHWAGANDHA: The Miraculous Herb! Holistic Solutions & Proven Healing Recipes for Health, Beauty, Weight Loss & Hormone Balance".

For now, Ashwagandha is just a guest in this recipe, not the main hero.

**Serves: 1-2**

**Ingredients:**

- 1 cup coconut milk
- Half cup fennel tea, cooled down
- 1 peach, peeled and pitted
- 1 banana, peeled and pitted
- Half teaspoon maca powder
- Half teaspoon Ashwagandha powder
- 1 inch ginger, peeled
- 1 teaspoon lemon juice, fresh
- Some ice cubes

**Instructions:**

1. Place all the ingredients in a blender.
2. Blend until creamy and smooth.
3. Drop in ice cubes and enjoy the creamy smoothie chilled.

## Recipe #29 Vitamin C Orange Smoothie

This recipe is just perfect if you are craving something sweet. It uses grapefruit and green tea. These are very helpful in weight loss and will help you stay energized. Green tea is also an amazing anti-oxidant.

**Serves: 1-2**

**Ingredients:**

- 1 whole orange, peeled and sliced
- 1 whole grapefruit, peeled and sliced
- 1 cup green tea, cooled down
- Half cup coconut water
- A handful of chopped pineapple

**Instructions:**

1. Place all the ingredients in a blender.
2. Process until smooth.
3. Drop a few ice cubes in the glass and serve right away.

## Recipe #30 Creamy Spinach Beauty Smoothie

Spinach, avocado and lemon juice is a unique combination. It offers a miraculous mix of energy boosting minerals such as magnesium, iron and calcium. You can use this smoothie as a meal replacement or even serve it as a warm soup.

You can add in some nuts, seeds or meat leftovers.

Who said that paleo cooking has to be complicated? It's the easiest eating system there is.

**Serves: 1**

**Ingredients:**

- 1 cup of fresh spinach leaves
- 1 whole avocado, pitted, peeled and diced
- 1 teaspoon of fresh lemon juice
- 1 cup of cashew milk
- Black pepper and Himalaya salt to taste
- Fresh cilantro leaves to garnish
- Optional: 2 small chili flakes if you like it spicy

**Instructions:**

1. Blend all the ingredients until smooth.
2. Serve as it is or chilled with ice cubes.
3. Enjoy!

## Recipe #31 Cherish Celery

This smoothie is full of the essential nutrients and vitamins like vitamin A, potassium, vitamin K2 and Vitamin B 6.

Coconut milk makes it very creamy and refreshing. It's also a perfect opportunity to add in some greens.

**Serves: 1-2**

**Ingredients:**

- ½ cup fresh cherries, pitted
- ½ cup of celery head
- A handful of spinach leaves, washed
- 2 tablespoons fresh mint leaves, one to add in to the smoothie, and one to garnish
- 1 cup of chilled coconut milk

**Instructions:**

1. Place all the ingredients and 1 tablespoon of fresh mint leaves in a blender.
2. Process until smooth.
3. Serve chilled with ice cubes and fresh mint leaves.
4. Enjoy!

## Recipe #32 Healthy Skin Smoothie

This smoothie combines the beta carotene of carrots and tomatoes. Drink this smoothie on a regular basis and you will have a healthy-looking skin. Turmeric and ginger add to anti-inflammatory properties. Grapefruit is full of Vitamin C and natural anti-oxidants.

One simple smoothie that combines so many superfoods, and all of them are easily accessible.

Plus, it tastes delicious and is very inexpensive to make.

**Serves: 1-2**

**Ingredients:**

- 1 cup of tomato, chopped and peeled
- ½ teaspoon of lemon juice
- 2 carrots
- 1 grapefruit, peeled
- 1 cup of water, filtered

**Instructions:**

1. Blend all the ingredients.
2. Serve the refreshing smoothie chilled.

## Recipe #33 Simple Nutty Paleo Protein Smoothie

This smoothie combines natural, plant-based protein with digestive and weight loss properties of fresh apples.

Paleo is not only about eating meat. It's also recommended to get some plant-based protein and eat some nuts and seeds.

Healthy eating is all about balance and this is exactly what we are trying to inspire though this book.

**Serves: 1-2**

**Ingredients:**

- 2 green apples, peeled, chopped and de-seeded
- A handful of walnuts, soaked for a few hours
- A handful of hazelnuts, soaked for a few hours
- 1 cup hazelnut milk
- 1 teaspoon nutmeg powder
- 1 teaspoon cinnamon powder

**Instructions:**

1. Blend all the ingredients.
2. Serve and enjoy.

## Recipe #34 Creamy Ginger Smoothie

Ginger is a very accessible superfood that very often gets overlooked.

The best way to use it is to add an inch or two to your smoothies.

Ginger adds to anti-inflammatory properties of your smoothies and it really tastes amazing. Enjoy!

**Serves: 1**

**Ingredients:**

- 1 apple, peeled
- 1 cup coconut milk
- 1 banana, peeled
- 1 inch ginger, peeled
- 1 peach, pitted
- Optional: 1 teaspoon moringa powder

**Instructions:**

1. Blend the apple and banana slices with coconut milk.
2. Add the peach and crushed ginger.
3. Drop in a few ice cubes, serve and enjoy.

## Part 2 Juices

Is juicing Paleo? Absolutely! These juices have a high concentration of zinc, calcium, iron, magnesium, phosphors, potassium, vitamins A, K, C, and E. They have lots of micronutrients, phytochemicals, chlorophyll and fiber.

While juicing can be a bit of a hussle and time-consuming, it's really worth it.
A 1 cup of fresh juice a day, or every other day is an excellent goal to begin with.

Health benefits of using Juices include:
- You give your digestive system a rest
- You get more energy
- It's easier to juice a mountain of fresh foods and veggies than to eat them
- Great for weight loss- you give your body a myriad of vitamins and nutrients with literally no calories. Your body gets hydrated and energized in a natural way and so you no longer crave unhealthy foods or sugars.

## Recipe #35 Cucumber Kale and Carrot Juice

Cucumber has 90% of water in them that plays an important role in breaking fat cells. Eating cucumber in plenty is wonderful since they are a natural procedure for weight loss.

While it's hard to eat a mountain of greens and cucumbers, it's easy to drink their juice and get all the vital nutrients in. Avocado oil offers good fat to help you absorb the minerals and vitamins from the juice.

**Servings: 2**

**Ingredients:**

- 2 big carrots, peeled and chopped
- 1 lemon, peeled
- 3 celery stalks, chopped
- A couple dashes of habanero hot sauce
- a handful of kale, chopped
- 2 big cucumbers, peeled and chopped
- a drizzle of avocado oil

**Instructions:**

1. Place through a juicer.
2. Juice.
3. Pour into a glass and add in a couple dashes of habanero hot sauce, if needed.

## Recipe #36 Flavored Spinach Juice

While pure spinach juice can be a bit hardcore, this recipe is a bit different. Add in some fresh apples and ginger and you will fall in love with green juice. One green juice a day will keep the doctor away!

**Serves: 2**

**Ingredients:**

- 2 cups of fresh spinach
- 2 green apples, peeled and chopped
- 2-inch ginger, peeled
- 1 tablespoon melted coconut oil

**Instructions:**

1. Place all the ingredients through a juicer.
2. Extract the juice, pour it in a big glass.
3. Add in some melted coconut oil.
4. Stir well and enjoy.

## Recipe #37 Watermelon Antioxidant Juice

Watermelon, ginger and healing greens is an excellent combination.

It makes the juice taste nice and helps you get accustomed to juicing greens.

**Servings: 2**

**Ingredients:**

- 1 cup of watermelon, chopped
- 1 cup mixed greens of your choice (I like to throw in some spinach, arugula and mint)
- 2 inch of ginger, peeled

**Instructions:**

5. Juice all the ingredients using a juicer.
6. Serve in a glass.
7. Enjoy!

## Recipe #38 Simple Apple Lemon Juice

Apples help maintain a healthy digestive system. Oh, and they make green juices taste great!

**Servings: 2**

**Ingredients:**

- 2 cups of kale, chopped
- 2 apples, peeled and chopped
- 1 lemon, peeled and halved
- 1 inch of ginger, peeled
- 1-inch turmeric, peeled

**Instructions:**

1. Place all the ingredients in a juicer.
2. Juice and serve in a glass.
3. Enjoy!

## Recipe #39 Honeydew Melon Green Juice

This is a super hydrating juice that combines the healing power of veggies and fruits. While a pure green juice may be a bit too much for a beginner, adding in some honeydew melon really takes it to a whole new level.

**Servings: 2**

**Ingredients:**

- 4 medium cucumbers, peeled and chopped
- 1 cup of honeydew melon
- 4 cup romaine lettuce

**Instructions:**

1. Place all the ingredients through a juicer.
2. Extract the juice.
3. Pour into a chilled glass and enjoy!

**Recipe #40 Easy Green Juice**

Red bell peppers are one of my favorite veggies to juice.

They are natural sweet and full of vitamins and minerals. They make any green juice taste amazing. Ginger adds to anti-inflammatory properties.

**Servings: 2**

**Ingredients:**

- 1 cup celery, chopped
- 3 red bell peppers, chopped
- 1 inch of ginger, peeled
- 2 slices of lime, to garnish
- Fresh ice cubes

**Instructions:**

1. Juice all the ingredients using a juicer.
2. Pour in a glass, add in some ice cubes.
3. Garnish with lime slices.
4. Serve and enjoy!

## Recipe #41 Coconut Kale Concoction

Compared to other juicing recipes, this one is relatively simple and quick to make as it leverages the coconut water. Just perfect as a quick, energy boosting juice

**Servings: 2**

**Ingredients:**

- 1 cup kale, chopped
- 1 green apple, cut into smaller pieces
- 1 cup of coconut water
- 1 teaspoon cinnamon powder

**Instructions:**

1. Juice the kale and apple.
2. Pour into a glass and mix with 1 cup of coconut water.
3. Stir well, add in 1 teaspoon of cinnamon powder and stir again.

## Recipe #42 Broccoli and Orange Juice

This juice is great for boosting your energy and stimulating weight loss.

It combines the healing and immune system boosting benefits of Vitamin C from oranges with the detoxifying properties of chlorophyll from the broccoli.

**Servings: 2**

**Ingredients:**

- 1 cup broccoli, chopped
- 4 oranges, peeled and cut into smaller pieces
- 1 lemon, peeled and cut into smaller pieces
- 1-½ cups of alkaline water

**Instructions:**

1. Place through a juicer.
2. Juice, and pour into a jar or a big glass and add in some water (you can skip this step if you like the intense taste of this juice)
3. Enjoy!

## Recipe #43 Green Tea High Energy Juice

This recipe is similar to the last one, however it also uses green tea to help you boost your energy levels and burn fat. Ginger adds to anti-inflammatory properties.

**Servings: 2**

**Ingredients:**

- 3 oranges, peeled and cut into smaller pieces
- Half cup spinach leaves
- 1 inch ginger, peeled
- 1 cup green tea, cooled down

**Instructions:**

1. Juice the oranges, ginger and spinach.
2. Pour into a glass or a jar and add in some green tea.
3. Enjoy!

## Recipe #44 A Beta Carotene Powerhouse

This juice is a fantastic combination of oranges, turmeric and carrots to help you have beautiful and healthy-looking skin while enjoying more energy without having to rely on caffeine.

**Servings: 2**

**Ingredients:**

- 6 carrots, peeled and chopped
- 2 oranges, peeled and cut into smaller pieces
- 1 lemon, peeled and cut into smaller pieces
- 1 zucchini, peeled and cut into smaller pieces
- 2-inch turmeric, peeled
- A few ice cubes (optional)
- A dash of cinnamon powder (optional)

**Instructions:**

1. Juice all the ingredients.
2. Pour into a glass and add in some ice cubes and a dash of cinnamon powder.
3. Enjoy!

## Recipe #45 A Restorative Antioxidant Juice

This juice is full of antioxidants and beta-carotene to help you have beautiful skin.

**Servings: 2**

**Ingredients:**

- 4 large Carrots, peeled and chopped
- 4 tomatoes, cut into smaller pieces
- 1 Garlic clove, peeled
- 1-inch ginger, peeled

**Instructions:**

1. Juice all the ingredients.
2. Pour into a glass and enjoy!

## Recipe #46 Veggie Medley Juice

Enjoy the wonderful mixture full of ingredients that make you healthy. They also contain antioxidant and elements that will help your body to fight against diseases and help in weight loss.

**Servings: 4**

**Ingredients:**

- 6 medium carrots, peeled and cut into smaller pieces
- 1 beet (with greens), peeled
- 3 large tomatoes, cut into smaller pieces
- 1 to 2 large handfuls spinach
- 1/8 head cabbage, chopped
- 3 kale leaves
- 1 red bell pepper, chopped
- 1 large celery stalk, chopped
- ¼ yellow onion, chopped
- ½ clove garlic, peeled
- ½ bunch parsley (optional)

**Instructions:**

1. Juice all the ingredients.
2. Pour into a glass.
3. If needed, season with some Himalaya salt.
4. Enjoy!

## Recipe #47 Cabbage and Coconut Juice

This recipe has plenty of antioxidants and is full of refreshing nutrients.

While pure green juice might be a bit too "hardcore" even for experienced juicing fanatics, it tastes amazing when mixed with other ingredients.

**Servings: 1**

**Ingredients:**

- ½ Cabbage, chopped
- ½ cup coconut water
- 4 green apples, chopped

**Instructions:**

1. Juice all the ingredients.
2. Pour into a glass and mix with some coconut water.
3. Enjoy!

## Recipe #48 Mixed Green Juice

This recipe is great if you happen to have some arugula leaves leftovers and don't feel like going for another salad. And yes, arugula juice tastes amazing when mixed with other ingredients!

**Servings: 2**

**Ingredients:**

- 1 cup arugula leaves
- A few pineapples slices
- 1 orange, peeled and cut into smaller pieces
- 1 lemon, peeled and cut into smaller pieces

**Instructions:**

1. Place though a juicer.
2. Juice and pour into a glass or a small jar.
3. Enjoy!

## Recipe #49 Tantalizing Green Juice

Once again, we are juicing arugula leaves while adding in some sweetness and vitamin C from Kiwis and anti-inflammatory benefits of ginger. Apple helps in digestion and lime adds even more of vitamin C and refreshing aroma.

**Servings: 2**

**Ingredients:**

- 1 cup arugula leaves
- 2 kiwis, peeled
- 1 green apple, cut into smaller pieces
- 1 lime, peeled and cut into smaller pieces
- 1-inch ginger, peeled

**Instructions:**

1. Place all the ingredients though a juicer.
2. Juice and enjoy!

**Recipe #50 Healing Carrot Juice**

Carrot juice tastes amazing and when combined with cucumber juice, it will help you stay hydrated and reduce unwanted sugar cravings for hours. Ashwagandha powder is optional here.

But it's a great choice to help you re-balance your energy levels while feeling more relaxed.

**Servings: 2**

**Ingredients:**

- 6 carrots, peeled and chopped
- 3 big cucumbers, peeled and chopped
- ¼ teaspoon Ashwagandha powder

**Instructions:**

1. Juice all the ingredients.
2. Pour into a glass and enjoy!

## Recipe #51 Cucumber's Delight

Cucumber contains water that provides a good environment for hydration and therefore contributes to weight loss. Parsley leaves add in a ton of vitamins and nutrients such as Vitamin A, Vitamin C and Iron. Mint helps in digestion and brings an amazing aroma to the table.

**Servings: 2**

**Ingredients:**

- 2 large cucumbers, peeled and chopped
- A handful of fresh mint leaves
- A handful of fresh parsley leaves

**Instructions:**

1. Juice all the ingredients.
2. Pour into a glass or a small jar.
3. Enjoy!

## Recipe #52 Turmeric Green Juice

Turmeric is full of polyphenols that help well in weight loss.

It's a great addition to your juices and creates a nice, spicy aroma that is very easy to get hooked on.

**Servings: 2**

**Ingredients:**

- 2 inch turmeric, peeled
- 2 inch ginger, peeled
- 2 oranges, peeled and cut into smaller pieces
- 1 lemon, peeled and cut into smaller pieces
- Half cup water, filtered

**Instructions:**

2. Juice all the ingredients.
3. Pour into a glass and mix with water.
4. Enjoy!

## Recipe #53 Pineapple Lime Mint Juice

This recipe balances the energy and weight loss stimulating benefits of greens with the sweetness of pineapple.

**Servings: 3-4**

**Ingredients:**

- ½ cup kale, chopped
- 1 cup pineapple, chopped
- ¼ cup mint leaves, fresh
- 2 limes, peeled and chopped

**Instructions:**

1. Place through a juicer.
2. Juice and pour into a glass.
3. Enjoy!

**Recipe #54 Orange Pomegranate Juice**

With Orange Pomegranate, you are sure of enjoying juice that is full of antioxidants and nutrients that are good for weight loss.

Oh, and we are snaking in some greens too. Great way to make use of some salad leftovers.

**Servings: 2**

**Ingredients:**

- 1 cup pomegranate seeds
- 1 cup of mixed greens of your choice
- 2 oranges, peeled and cut into smaller pieces

**Instructions:**

1. Place through a juicer.
2. Pour into a glass and enjoy!

## Recipe #55 Coconut Flavored Green Juice

The ingredients are rich in phytonutrients and antioxidants. The juice relaxes the body and makes it easy to lose extra pounds.

**Servings: 2**

**Ingredients:**

- 1 cup kale, chopped
- 2 tablespoons coconut oil
- 1 cup pineapple, chopped
- 1 green apple, chopped

**Instructions:**

1. Place all the ingredients through a juicer.
2. Juice and pour into a glass
3. Enjoy!

# Part 3 Teas and Herbal Infusions

When you mention the word *detoxification*, you can't miss the benefits of tea.

Black and green teas have antioxidants in them, good for the detoxification process and alleviating the risks of chronic inflammation. Herbal tea contains infusions that comprise of spices and herbs and does not contain caffeine.

Tea is good for flushing out unwanted toxins from your body and has the capacity to cut down on the fat cells too.

You've probably heard of Chinese men and women living well past the 100-year mark. Most of them attribute their long life to drinking tea. They consume the tea on a daily basis and drink 2-3 times a day.

Tea helps to boost your energy as well. It's the caffeine that helps in increasing your energy and keeping you fit. You will have enough energy to last throughout a busy day. If you wake up feeling out of sorts, a refreshing cup of tea can chase the blues away and lighten your mood.

If you suffer from insomnia or have trouble sleeping, then herbal tea can help to solve the problem. By consuming chamomile tea on a regular basis, you can effectively eliminate the problem and fall asleep much more easily. Apart from chamomile, there are also other concoctions that you can brew and consume to fall asleep better.

We will look at these teas in the following recipes.

## Recipe #56 Ginger and Turmeric Tea

This tea is great for getting rid of coughs and colds and will perform wonders for those looking to lose excess weight.

**Serves: 1**

**Ingredients:**

- 1 inch ginger, peeled
- 1 inch turmeric, peeled
- 1 cup water, boiling
- 1 Indian spice blend tea bag
- 1 teaspoon honey

**Instructions:**

1. Place all the tea ingredients (except honey) in a tea pot and pour over some boiling water.
2. Keep covered for 15 minutes.
3. Strain and serve warm (but not boiling) in a tea cup with 1 teaspoon of honey.

*Note: If you are unable to find the Indian spice tea bags then you can prepare your own. To prepare the tea bag mix together tea leaves along with a couple of cloves, 1 black cardamom pod, 1 teaspoon black pepper corns, ½ inch cinnamon stick and a few green cardamom pods.*

## Recipe #57 Easy Chili Tea

This tea will help in cleansing your digestive tract while warming you up and giving you a strong energy boost that will last for hours.

**Serves: 2**

**Ingredients:**

- 2 cups water, boiling.
- 2 green tea bags
- 2 red chili flakes
- A handful of fresh mint leaves
- 2 tablespoons honey

**Instructions:**

1. Place all the tea ingredients (except honey) in a tea pot and pour over 2 cups of boiling water.
2. Keep covered for 15 minutes.
3. Strain and serve warm (but not boiling) in a tea cup with 1 teaspoon of honey.

## Recipe #58 Cumin and Caraway Tea

This tea is great for those women looking to obtain relief from period cramps.

**Serves: 1-2**

**Ingredients:**

- 2 cups water, boiling
- 1 black tea bag (optional, if you need an energy boost but you can skip it if you want to keep it 100% caffeine-free)
- 1 inch ginger, peeled
- 1 tablespoon cumin seeds
- 1 tablespoon caraway seeds
- 1 tablespoon coriander seeds
- 1 tablespoon fennel seeds
- 1 tablespoon honey, if needed

**Instructions:**

1. Place all the tea ingredients (except honey) in a tea pot and pour over 2 cups of boiling water.
2. Keep covered for 15 minutes.
3. Strain and serve warm (but not boiling) in a tea cup with 1 teaspoon of honey.

## Recipe #59 Spicy Chai Tea

This tea is super tasty and creamy. It can be consumed on a regular basis and it's great to prevent colds too.

**Serves: 1-2**

**Ingredients:**

- 1 cup almond or coconut milk
- 1 Indian chai tea bag
- 2 inch turmeric, peeled
- 2 tablespoons honey

**Instructions:**

1. Boil almond milk using a saucepan
2. When boiling, add the tea bag and turmeric.
3. Simmer on low heat for 5 minutes.
4. Turn off the heat and keep covered for 15 minutes.
5. Pour into a tea cup and sweeten with honey if needed

In the absence of chai tea, make use of tea leaves mixed with cinnamon, cloves and cardamon Make it sweet and healthy by adding the almond milk.

## Recipe #60 Ashwagandha Tea

This is a great tea for those looking to boost their sex drive. It is also good for those looking to increase their immunity.

**Serves: 1-2**

**Ingredients:**
- 1 tablespoon dried ashwagandha
- 2 cups water, boiling
- 1 fennel tea bag
- 1 green tea bag
- 1 tablespoon honey (optional)

**Instructions:**
1. Place all the tea ingredients (except honey) in a tea pot and pour over some boiling water.
2. Keep covered for 15 minutes.
3. Strain and serve warm (but not boiling) in a tea cup with 1 teaspoon of honey (if needed)

## Recipe #61 Sleep Well Tea

This recipe will help you unwind after a busy day, sleep like a baby and wake up feeling energized.

**Serves: 2**

**Ingredients**

- 1 cup of water, boiling
- 1 lemongrass stalk
- 2 tablespoons chamomile tea
- A few tablespoons of coconut milk
- 1 tablespoon of coconut oil
- A dash of cinnamon powder to garnish

**Instructions:**

1. Place all the tea ingredients (except coconut milk and oil) in a tea pot and pour over some boiling water.
2. Keep covered for 15 minutes.
3. Strain.
4. Pour into a tea cup and add in the coconut milk and oil.
5. Stir well.
6. Sprinkle over some cinnamon powder, enjoy!

## Bonus Recipe: Easy Mediterranean Tea

*This tea can be made in 2 different ways:*

1.You can choose to add in some green tea, if you need more energy, for example if you are using this tea in the morning.

2.You can choose to add in some Melissa tea, if you need to unwind, for example if you are using this tea in the evening and want to unwind and sleep well.

Rosemary and fennel are both miraculous herbs and will help you boost your immune system and fight off colds and flu.

Fennel is also great for weight loss as well as stimulating your lymphatic system.

**Serves: 2**

**Ingredients:**

- 2 cups boiling water
- 1 tablespoon rosemary herb
- 1 tablespoon fennel seeds
- 1 teaspoon green tea, or Melissa tea (optional)

**Instructions:**

1. Place all the tea ingredients (except honey) in a tea pot and pour over some boiling water.
2. Keep covered for 15 minutes.
3. Strain and serve warm (but not boiling) in a tea cup with 1 teaspoon of honey (if needed)

# Bonus Recipe: Lime Refresher Ice Tea

Blueberries are known for their anti-oxidant providing abilities and they are wonderfully sweet. Add the addition of spicy herb and a lime twist, and you have a hydrating drink that is fully paleo!

### Ingredients

- 2 cups of blueberries
- 2 limes
- 1 medium bunch of fresh oregano
- 1 liter of water – filtered if liked

### Instructions

1. Pour the water in to a suitable container or jug.
2. Wash the blueberries and limes.
3. Add the blueberries to the water, squashing a third of them on to a plate beforehand, and catching any juice to add too.
4. Juice one of the limes and add the juice to the water. Slice the other lime in to thin pieces.
5. Wash the oregano and give it a bit of a "squeeze" to start releasing some of it's flavor.
6. Add the herbs to the water and mix really well. Leave in the fridge for at least an hour before serving.

## Final Words and Your Paleo Quick Start Guide

We hope you enjoyed the recipes and feel inspired to live a Paleo lifestyle.

We are adding this short Paleo guide to help you on your health journey.

Remember, it's not about being perfect. Even if you do Paleo "part time", but you listen to your body and focus on adding as many healthy foods as possible, you are good to go.

It's not about going hungry or getting too caught up in counting calories.

## Paleo Lifestyle Made Easy

The Paleo diet is an approach to eating that originated a long time ago, during the Paleolithic era. This time frame started about 2.5 million years ago and ended around 10,000 years before our time. It avoids eating foods that only became part of the human diet after the agricultural revolution. The idea is that diseases like cancer and diabetes started around the same time that we began growing our own foods. The underlying principle is that the hunter-gatherers' diet is the reason they did not develop such diseases.

While we cannot be sure that their diet is what kept them healthy, there is enough research that concludes that foods banned from Paleo diets have little or no beneficial nutritional value. They have also been proven to interrupt normal hormonal balances, cause inflammation, and damage the lining of the gut. Eating Paleo will help to balance our bodies internally, protect the kidneys, protect the digestive tract from destructive proteins like gluten, and keep the liver and pancreas from having to work too hard.

Many names and titles have been given to this age-old eating program: the Paleolithic diet, Paleolithic nutrition, Paleo diet, Stone Age diet, caveman diet, and hunter-gatherer diet. Paleo Diet is an effort to go back to eating how we were biologically intended to eat. This method enables us to fuel our bodies properly so that they may function at their full genetic potential and start living healthier immediately. Foods that could be collected and consumed by hunting and gathering are what need to focus on. Primal eating at its best.

For me, I like to think of it as a Paleo perspective, not an actual diet. It could also be called a template. However you look at it, it is a lifestyle change. The goal is to eat like our ancestors did millions of years ago before the Agricultural Revolution.

Here are seven guidelines for Paleo nutrition that helped me to get a better idea of the principles involved in this primal nutritional practice.

1. **Increase protein intake.**

15% of the calories in most diets are from protein. When adhering to Paleo, that percentage must be much higher. It should be between 19-35 percent. A large amount of animal protein is required.

2. **Decrease carbohydrate intake and eat foods lower on the glycemic index.**

Most of the carbs will come from vegetables (and a few fruits). They should take up between 35-45 percent of your daily caloric intake. Most of the foods you will eat will be low on the glycemic index. They will not make your blood sugar spike because they are assimilated slowly.

3. **Increase fiber consumption.**

Paleos get their fiber from non-starchy vegetables. Vegetables such as these usually contain a fiber content around 30 percent higher than processed grain and about eight times higher than whole grain. Even fruits have more fiber than whole and refined grains.

4. **Increase fat intake by eating more monounsaturated and polyunsaturated fats.**

You need to do this in combination with a good balance of Omega-3 and Omega-6 fats. It is a common misconception that health is related to how *much* fat you eat, when the *type* of fat you eat affects your health more. Increase monounsaturated and Omega-3 fats and remove Trans and Omega-6 polyunsaturated fats.

5. **Raise potassium while lowering sodium.**

Paleolithic humans consumed foods that were unrefined and fresh. Potassium levels in fresh foods are between 5-10 percent higher than sodium levels. Potassium helps the heart, kidneys, and other organs function correctly. People who have low potassium levels are more susceptible to elevated blood pressure, stroke, and cardiovascular disease. Excessive sodium levels can also cause the same problems. Many modern diets contain two times as much sodium as potassium.

6. **Eat more alkaline than acidic foods.**

When we consume food, it has either an acid or alkaline effect on your body. Even on a Paleo diet, it is necessary to keep this in mind because meat and fish are both acid-forming foods. Alkaline-producing foods include most vegetables and fruits. Having an acidic system for a long time can lead to atrophy of the muscles and bone, elevated blood pressure, kidney stones, and can trigger things like asthma and allergies.

7. **Increase the intake of vitamins, phytochemicals, minerals, and antioxidants.**

Whole grains are a poor source of these things. The few minerals and vitamins that are actually in whole grains are not usually processed and absorbed properly by the body. They do not contain vitamin C, A, or B12. There truly is no substitute for grass-produced and free-range meat or organic vegetables and fruits.

What foods did the cavemen eat? What foods did they hunt, and what did they go out and gather? These are two key questions to keep in mind when deciding what to eat on the Paleo diet.

**Basic categories of foods to consume when eating Paleo:**

- Grass-produced meats
- Fish and seafood

- Eggs
- Fresh fruits and vegetables
- Seeds
- Healthful oils (olive, walnut, flaxseed, macadamia, avocado, or coconut)

The foods included on the Paleo diet are foods that our cave-dwelling ancestors would have access to on a regular basis.

Basic categories of what NOT to eat when eating Paleo:
- Cereals and grains
- Potatoes
- Legumes
- Sugars
- Processed foods
- Salt
- Dairy
- Refined vegetable oil

Some people do not understand exactly what a legume is. A legume is the seed pod of a plant that is edible. Examples of legumes are:
- Beans
- Peas
- Lentils
- Soy

Essentially, if a caveman could not have eaten it 10,000 years ago, you cannot eat it now. No consuming packaged foods at all. If it contains chemicals or ingredients that you cannot pronounce, then it is probably not Paleo.

Inflammation is the body's natural response to invaders. I already discussed this problem and how "leaky gut" will lead to weight gain. It may be more important to note that "leaky gut" will lead to major health issues because it causes chronic inflammation. Cancer, asthma, headaches, allergies, arthritis, auto-immune disorders, heart disease, diabetes, depression, Alzheimer's, and osteoporosis are all caused by chronic inflammation. The list goes on and on.

Why does inflammation cause so many problems? Inflammation is an immune system response. It is used by the body to battle intruders that are unidentified or already deemed harmful. Well, how could something good cause such a problem? Let me explain it this way. It is like leaving the heater turned up and the thermostat not working. It never turns off when the environment gets to a certain temperature. Yes, you wanted to warm up, but if it never turns off, it will get way too hot. It will negatively affect whatever is in the environment.

Converting to a Paleolithic nutritional lifestyle has allowed me to eat a diet that is void of inflammatory foods. Aside from healing "leaky gut," thus allowing the immune system to calm down, Paleo diets also reduce inflammation in many other ways. I have highlighted a few below:

- The diet is high in vitamin D. Vitamin D has been proven to aid in reducing inflammation.

- The diet is high in phytonutrients, many of which have anti-inflammatory effects.

- The immune system reacts to factors in the environment that it has been exposed to (pollen, bacteria, molds, etc.) with inflammation. The Paleo diet has the effect of making the immune system less prone to react to these factors and also makes it more effective because it is not over-loaded.

- The Paleo perspective adjusts the Omega-3/Omega-6 proportion to a beneficial ratio and makes it an effective agent in battling inflammatory illnesses. An Omega-3/6 imbalance can result from eating vegetable oils, grain products, and a deficiency of DHA and EPA from animal products.

Reading labels is a must-do for any Paleo dieter. For the most part, anything with a label is probably something you do not want to buy. If it does have a label, but you can't pronounce the ingredients, do not purchase it. Here are some things that I keep in mind when I grocery shop:

Best = Zero ingredients

Better = One ingredient

Ok = Two ingredients

Pushing my luck = Three ingredients

No way = Four+ ingredients

**Key words to remember when shopping to stock a Paleo kitchen**: Organic, grass-fed, pasture-raised, wild-caught, free-range, and raw.

I had to replace everything in my pantry with new ingredients that I would be using in Paleo recipes. I had previewed these new recipes, and if you are anything like me, these ingredients sounded strange. They are staples of the Paleo kitchen and will benefit you in preparing many delicious Paleo meals and snacks. This a list of items that are usually used in Paleo recipes:

- **Blanched almond flour**

- **Coconut flour**

- **Almond meal**

- **Extra virgin coconut Oil**

- **Refined coconut oil**

- **Palm shortening**

- **Arrowroot powder/Tapioca starch**

- **Ground flax meal**

- **Coconut milk**

- **Creamed coconut**

- Unsweetened coconut flakes

- Unsweetened shredded coconut

- Nuts: Whole almonds, pecan halves, walnut halves, macadamia nuts, hazelnuts, pistachios, cashews, Brazil nuts

- Almond Butter

- Raw/natural cocoa powder

- Honey

- Raw maple syrup

- Leavening/Spices: Baking soda, cream of tartar, allspice, cinnamon, salt, cloves, cardamom, ground ginger, nutmeg, vanilla extract, vanilla bean, lemon juice

**We Need Your Help**

One more thing, before you go, could you please do us a quick favor?

It would be great if you could leave us a short review on Amazon.

Don't worry, it doesn't have to be long. One sentence is enough.

Let others know your favorite recipes and who you think this book can help.

You will find similar books and other resources to help you on your weight loss and wellness journey at:

www.YourWellnessBooks.com

www.ingramcontent.com/pod-product-compliance
Lightning Source LLC
Chambersburg PA
CBHW081409080526
44589CB00016B/2506